Understanding Allergies

Understanding Allergies

Mary Steel

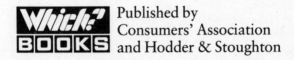 Published by
Consumers' Association
and Hodder & Stoughton

Understanding Allergies is published in Great Britain by
Consumers' Association, 14 Buckingham Street, London WC2N 6DS
and Hodder & Stoughton, 47 Bedford Square, London WC1B 3DP

First Edition
Copyright © 1986 Consumers' Association

British Library Cataloguing in Publication Data

Steel, Mary
    Understanding allergies.
    1. Allergy
    I. Title   II. Consumers' Association
    616.97   RC584

ISBN 0-340-38162-0

Typographic design by Tim Higgins
Cover illustration and cartoons by John Holder
Photoset in Great Britain by Rowland Phototypesetting Ltd
Bury St Edmunds, Suffolk
Printed and bound in Great Britain by
Garden City Press, Letchworth, Herts

Contents

Introduction

Allergies may well be as old as man himself. Evidence of their ancient history, recorded by great physicians thousands of years ago, is given in the following chapter. Yet the word allergy did not even exist before this century.

It was used for the first time in 1906 as a composite of two Greek words, 'allos' meaning altered and 'ergon', reaction. The meaning of allergy is therefore 'altered capacity to react'. It is only in the last two or three decades, as advanced science and technology have revealed the awesome complexities of the immune system, that it has been possible to understand something of what occurs in allergic reaction.

Well-recognised diseases such as hay fever and asthma are now known to be the result of hypersensitivity, a malfunction of the immune system. A multitude of substances, harmless to the majority of people, trigger the system into activity, producing many different symptoms according to what part of the body is affected.

The efficiency of the immune system is crucial to man's survival as a species. The devastation which occurs when it breaks down, as opposed to when it malfunctions, can be seen in the present world-wide outbreak of the viral disease AIDS (acquired immune deficiency syndrome). Victims die most often from lung infections or cancer because the virus seriously impairs the immune function.

It is not only in the context of AIDS that immunology is referred to constantly in newspapers and on television. It plays a vital role in organ transplants when a patient must take drugs to suppress the immune system to prevent its rejecting the new heart or kidney. It has been observed that transplant victims run an increased risk of developing cancer as a result. This supports the theory of 'immune surveillance' – that in a healthy individual pre-cancerous cells are constantly identified by the immune system and destroyed before malignancy develops.

Compared with the dire effects of impaired immunity, the hypersensitivity which leads to allergic reactions may seem hardly more than an inconvenience. Yet deaths to occur – principally from asthma – despite the formidable armoury of medication now available. And all sufferers from allergic disorders will testify to the misery and disruption of normal life they cause.

The word allergy was born with the century and indeed the present decade has seen the whole field expand so that there seems no disease more fashionable or word more misused. The increased interest in food and nutrition has given an extra impetus to the theories of the clinical ecologists. Starting in the USA, this movement believes that allergy resulting from modern food and environmental factors may be responsible for many illnesses outside the accepted group of classical allergies.

Confusion, misinformation and controversy cloud the issues. Statistical evidence regarding allergies is notoriously uneven because of the lack of internationally recognised criteria for studies. An incidence of one person in three suffering from some form of allergy in industrialised countries is suggested by some authorities – others put it even higher and bidding to surpass infection as a cause of illness.

The importance of the field was recognised by the World Health Organisation when it called a conference in 1984 to discuss the prevention of allergies. Some material presented there is included in these pages.

This book makes a limited use of medical terms and unfamiliar words can be found in the glossary on page 162. One such word, originating in the 1920s, probably sums up the whole curious world of allergies with its many remaining mysteries. An adjective to describe the illnesses and those who suffer from them is 'atopic'. It means strange or out of place (from Greek 'topos': place).

I

The history of allergy

References to what we now know as allergies stretch back into antiquity. Asthma and food allergies were the main allergic conditions to feature in the observations of the earliest physicians – not surprisingly, because both can be grave, occasionally even fatal. In contrast, the sneezing of hay fever and the itch of eczema or urticaria would have seemed trivialities to doctors faced daily with smallpox, leprosy and syphilis, all well documented in ancient times.

Not all the earliest references were written. One of these exceptions, more haunting than any description, is a figurine found in Mexico, dated about AD 400 and owned by Glaxo in the USA. The tiny figure sits hunched on the ground, legs crossed and arms folded in agony across his chest. His face is contorted, the mouth a panting gape. Nobody who has ever suffered or witnessed a severe attack of asthma could fail to recognise the cause of his misery.

Asthma in adults and children was recognised by Hippocrates (460 BC – circa 359 BC), 'the Father of Medicine' who is remembered today every time a student entering the medical profession takes the Hippocratic oath. He recorded the spasmodic nature of the illness and suggested cold as one precipitating factor, an observation confirmed by modern medicine.

He also recognised food allergy, writing that although cheese was an excellent food for most men, some were made ill by the smallest piece. In seeking the cause of disease, Hippocrates was deeply concerned about food. Similarly, he laid great stress upon the importance of occupation and climate, both highly relevant to the diagnosis of allergies.

The words 'asthma' and 'eczema' were both in use in his lifetime. The first comes from the Greek root which means 'panting', the second meaning 'bubble, boil, burst forth'. No doubt asthma was then what it remains today, one of the most wretched and debilitating illnesses. 'Eczema', however, was used much less specifically and could refer to many different skin eruptions.

Many of the most ancient treatments foreshadowed modern approaches to breathing difficulties. The Ebers Papyrus, dating from about 1550 BC and named after the Egyptologist who discovered it, recommended an inhalation of herbs. Much later the Greek physician Galen (AD 130–AD 201), regarded as second to Hippocrates, advised his Roman patients suffering from asthma to climb Mount Etna and breathe the sulphurous fumes of the volcano.

Ancient herbal manuals contain recommendations for inhalations to relieve asthma, including drugs which have stood the test of time. In China, a catalogue of medicinal plants traditionally dates from the twenty-eighth century BC when the semi-mythical emperor Shen Nung listed 365 species. This included ephedrine (used to treat asthma), which was obtained from a native Chinese shrub, was later grown in India and introduced into Britain in the late nineteenth century. Early this century herbal cigarettes were a popular form of treatment for asthmatics.

The Assyrian Herbal included deadly nightshade as a treatment for asthma. This plant is also native to England and Wales where its dull purple flowers and black berries can be seen in woods and thickets. Its poisonous properties are common knowledge. Modern pharmacologists recognise that it is the presence of atropine in the plant which makes it an effective drug. Both ephedrine and atropine are still in limited use for the treatment of asthma today although unlike the modern drug, sodium cromoglycate, they are banned under Olympic rules.

Even in Roman times it was known that the emotions

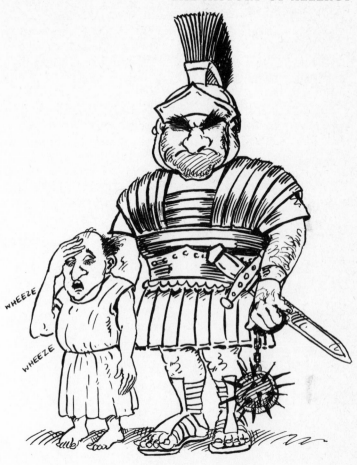

could play a part in the onset of an attack of asthma. Sufferers were not subjected to torture because it had been observed that wheezing, induced by fear, would make them unable to speak a word.

Lacking even the simplest tools of science, the ancient physicians had to rely upon keen observation of their patients. They wrote meticulously accurate descriptions of disease which are often difficult to better. One example is

11

the description of an attack of asthma by the Greek Aretaeus who lived in Rome in the second half of the second century AD. He spoke of the early symptoms as a feeling of weight on the chest, an unwillingness to attend to ordinary business and difficulty in breathing when running or going uphill.

Later, patients were affected with hoarseness and coughing, 'the nose sharp and greedy of air'. He went on that the voice was feeble, indicating the presence of mucus, and that patients could not lie down but preferred to sit up in order to draw in all the air possible.

The modern allergist needs the same power of observation and enquiry as the ancient physician. Detailed investigation always forms the basis for diagnosis of allergies although modern science now provides a whole range of laboratory facilities to reinforce case histories.

Hippocrates recorded the allergenic effect of cheese. Before long strawberries, nuts, shellfish and eggs were added to the list. Doctors were beginning to pick up strange unrelated clues to a puzzle that would take many centuries even to begin to solve.

As well as observing and treating allergies, ancient physicians employed the principles of the overall science of immunology. Centuries before 1798 when Edward Jenner published his discovery that vaccination with cowpox produced immunity from smallpox (see below), the Chinese were practising a form of immunisation against the same disease – 'the flowers of heaven'. Their method was to take crusts from pustules of sufferers with a mild form of the disease. These crusts were then ground to a powder and sniffed up the nose as a preventative.

Early in the eighteenth century, Lady Mary Wortley Montagu, wife of a British ambassador to the court of Constantinople, introduced a Turkish method of immunisation to Britain. Variolation, as it was known, was practised by using a large needle – 'no more than a scratch,' said Lady Mary – and introducing matter from a smallpox pustule. Having lost a brother to the disease, Lady Mary had her own small son treated in 1717. Although the practice became quite widespread and was legalised in France in 1755, it failed to control the terrible incidence of the disease.

According to legend, some individuals also discovered the secret of immunity to poison. One story concerns Mithridates VI, or the Great (132 BC–63 BC), king of Pontus. His attempt to conquer all Asia Minor led to war with Rome in 88 BC. Mithridates had a deep fear of poison, a common weapon of the time. He is said to have dosed himself with small and then gradually increasing doses of poisons until he became immune to their effects.

There is an ironical twist to this grim tale. Faced with complete defeat by the Roman Pompey, Mithridates decided upon suicide and had to order one of his mercenaries to despatch him with a sword. However, he is said to have successfully poisoned several of his wives and children.

This story encourages speculation about another death many centuries later, the murder of Rasputin in 1916. The leader of the assassins, Prince Yussupov, later attested that Rasputin seemed to be invulnerable to poison which was the first method employed to kill him. It seems possible that Rasputin, fearing for his life (with good reason), had taken the same precautions as Mithridates.

During medieval times, there were no great advances in medicine and the judgements of the towering figures of the past, Hippocrates and Galen for example, remained unchallenged.

With the Renaissance, however, there came a change of direction in the study of medicine. Instead of accepting the precepts of the past, students turned to anatomy and physiology and became equipped to define diseases more scientifically.

The reputation of some doctors spread far beyond their own countries. This was the reason why the Scottish Archbishop of St Andrews, John Hamilton, who lived in the sixteenth century, was able to consult an Italian physician, Jerome Cardan of Pavia (1501–1576). The Archbishop suffered from severe asthma and, apparently dissatisfied with local doctors, sent for Cardan who travelled to Scotland to treat him. Cardan's treatment was not lengthy. He advised the Archbishop to get rid of the feather quilt and pillows on his bed. Feathers are well known today as a common allergen. Taking Cardan's advice, the Archbishop made such a rapid recovery that he rewarded Cardan with 1,400 gold pieces and a gold chain to wear round his neck. The perceptive Cardan was one of an increasing number of doctors who noted allergic cause and effect without the slightest idea of the physiological process which linked them.

Hay fever made its first recorded appearance in the sixteenth century curiously disguised as 'rose fever'. The disorder was characterised by itching of the nose, sneezing and a headache, familiar symptoms to modern sufferers. However, it is now known that hay fever is not caused by pollen from colourful flowers like roses. Garden flowers have heavy sticky pollen and rely upon insects for pollination. Allergists now believe that rose fever was caused by grass pollens that settled on the petals of roses while they were in bloom.

In Italy about the same time, the physician Pietro Mattioli (1500–1577) reported the symptoms of a patient suffering from 'cat fever'. Cats are now known as a very common source of allergic reaction. Mattioli's patient suffered agitation, sweating and pallor in the presence of a cat and reacted in the same way even if the cat was concealed from him. It is likely that the 'agitation' marked the early signs of breathing difficulties which can be provoked by the dander (skin particles) of many animals.

The first observation of allergy to a drug was made in the middle of the seventeenth century when the Portuguese introduced the ipecacuanha root from Brazil. Used to induce vomiting, the root was also effective in smaller doses as an aid to digestion and an expectorant. Before long some pharmacists discovered that they developed eye irritation and breathing difficulties while pounding the root to make the medicine. A few were so severely affected that they could not even remain in the same room as a colleague working with ipecacuanha. This root is in use in the pharmaceutical industry today and some workers still complain of its effects.

Baker's asthma was recognised as early as 1700. The explanation then proposed by doctors, although plausible at the time, looks quaint in retrospect. They believed that the breathing difficulties suffered by some bakers were due to their drawing tiny pieces of dough into their lungs. It is now known that the cause does lie with the raw materials in a bakehouse, but is due to an allergic reaction either to flour

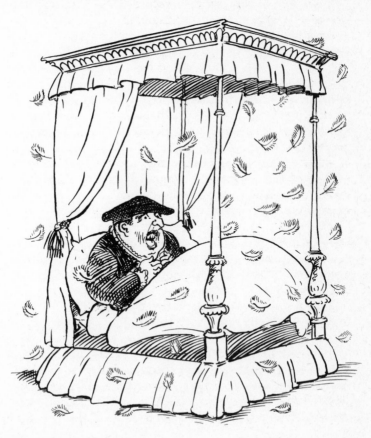

or to yeast, a type of mould, the spores of which are easily inhaled; or it can be caused by the wheat weevil which contaminates the flour.

Early pioneers each made a contribution to the vast jigsaw of allergic reaction. Dr William Cullen (1710–1790), a Professor of Medicine at both Glasgow and Edinburgh Universities, was the first to use the word 'idiosyncrasy' where today we would say 'allergy'. It was not at all a bad word to use. The *Concise Oxford Dictionary* gives one meaning as 'physical constitution peculiar to a person'. He observed that patients suffering from idiosyncrasies, often hereditary, suffered ill effects – pain and sickness for example – after eating certain foods. He listed white of egg, honey, milk and shellfish as examples of those foods, all of them already noted by the ancient Greeks.

The sting of a bee or wasp was the subject of medical record for the first time in France in 1765. Dr Desbret, a graduate of the University of Montpellier with a country practice near Vichy, described the death of a farmer from a bee sting. The man was working in his garden in mid-April when he was stung on the temple by a bee. He immediately fell to the ground and died within minutes.

Towards the end of the eighteenth century, Edward Jenner's discovery of vaccination as a protection against smallpox set the scene for the development of immunology as an important science. The earlier practice of variolation had not worked. It was, at best, a hit and miss method and those treated often passed the disease on to others. In the eighteenth century, it has been reckoned that 16 out of every 100 Londoners were pockmarked. They were the lucky ones for the disease was often fatal.

Edward Jenner (1749–1823) had studied under the great surgeon John Hunter at St George's Hospital, London, and then practised for the rest of his life in Gloucestershire. From 1775 Jenner made a study of cowpox, noting that while dairymaids often had lesions of the disease on their hands, they seemed to be immune to smallpox. In 1796 he successfully inoculated an eight-year-old boy from the cowpox lesions of a dairymaid. Two years later his famous paper was published on the first successful case of vaccination (from the Latin 'vacca': cow). Jenner's discovery eventually rid the world of the scourge of smallpox.

With the coming of the nineteenth century a phenomenon typical of the field of allergy made an appearance – the physician who was also a patient. One of the first of many advances made by doctors who were also sufferers was achieved by the London physician John Bostock (1773–1846). In 1819 he read a paper to the Royal Medical Chirurgical Society entitled: 'Case of periodical affection of the eyes and chest'. The patient, of course, was Bostock. His paper gave the first clinical description of hay fever. Nine years later he described 18 additional cases and proposed that the disease be called 'summer catarrh'. He did not really think that new-mown hay had anything to do with his symptoms which he was inclined to blame on sunshine and warmth. However, the general opinion among sufferers was that it all began with hay, and as 'fever' then simply meant ailment and not heightened temperature as it does now, 'hay fever' was quickly accepted as the name of the new illness.

It was not until the latter part of the century that a Mancunian, Charles Harrison Blackley (1820–1900), demonstrated that pollen could cause hay fever. Regarded as a crank by many of his contemporaries, Blackley was a homoeopath who did not begin studying medicine until he was 35. Like Bostock, he was a hay fever sufferer. He was also a man of original mind with a facility for devising ingenious experiments, and made hundreds of tests on himself with many other materials such as dust as well as a variety of pollens.

Having decided that pollens caused hay fever, Blackley set about determining the concentration of pollen in the atmosphere. He moistened glass slides with glycerine to catch pollen grains and so demonstrated that his patients' symptoms worsened when the air was heavily charged with pollen. He mounted his slides on kites which rose to heights

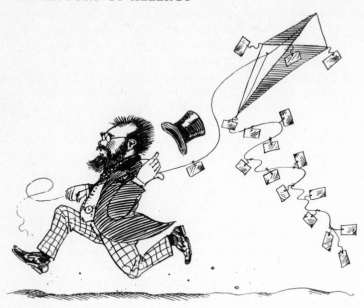

of 500 metres and found plenty of pollen there. He speculated, for that was all he could do, about the possible presence of pollen in the upper atmosphere beyond his reach. We now know that pollen can be blown to great heights.

As well as anticipating the modern method used to obtain a pollen count, Blackley described an experiment in which he obtained a positive reaction to pollen with a scratch test on his forearm. The method he used was very similar to the modern scratch test for allergens. Having abraded both forearms with a lancet, he applied pollen grains on a piece of wet lint to one abrasion only. No pollen was introduced to the other arm.

Only a few minutes after the pollen had been applied, the spot began to itch intensely and the parts around the abrasion began to swell. The swelling continued until there was a weal six centimetres long resembling what is now known as urticaria. Blackley had discovered a cause of the weal and flare reaction. The arm to which no pollen had been applied produced no swelling or irritation.

The science of immunology also burgeoned in the nineteenth century under the direction of such men as Louis Pasteur (1822–1895). He discovered how to immunise humans and dogs against rabies, sheep and cattle against anthrax (which could be transmitted to people) and fowl against chicken cholera. Antivenin was also developed for snake bites by the classical method of injecting horses with snake venom and then preparing a horse serum for injection into a human patient.

Pierre Roux (1853–1933), Pasteur's first assistant who later became director of the Pasteur Institute in Paris, was responsible for the production of diphtheria antitoxin. He was the first man to propose that an invading bacillus or germ produced poison or toxin in the patient.

It also became clear that immunity against toxin could be gained if the body was stimulated to produce antibodies against it. Johannes Müller had been the first physician to use the microscope in 1830 and this invaluable tool was to play a vital role in revealing the linked mysteries of allergy and immunology. While still a student, the brilliant Paul Ehrlich (1854–1915) identified the mast cell in connective tissue for the first time. It is now known that this particular cell is an important link in the chain of allergic reaction (see Chapter 2).

Twentieth-century discoveries

Just after the turn of the century, Charles Richet, Professor of Physiology at the University of Paris, began a series of studies with the then Prince of Monaco, grandfather of Prince Rainier. The prince was an outstanding ocean-ographer and put his scientifically equipped yacht at the disposal of Richet. The object of the research was to produce immunity to poison in test dogs by injecting repeated small doses over a period of weeks. The experiment recalled exactly the legend of Mithridates 2,000 years earlier.

Richet's first trials were made with poison from the deadly Portuguese man-of-war, a jellyfish which plagues the Mediterranean. He later turned to the comparatively harmless sea anemone. One of his subjects was 'a fine big dog by the name of Neptune'. Three weeks after his first injection of poison, Neptune was given a second measuring only one-tenth of a fatal dose, but within a few seconds the dog was extremely ill and soon fell dead.

This seemed to confound all the premises already established about acquired immunity. What was at first an apparently harmless substance had become deadly. Richet and his junior colleague Portier had stumbled upon the principle of anaphylaxis (see Chapter 9), a word they created to express the opposite of prophylaxis, meaning protection.

After further experiments, Richet made a report with his colleague and the importance of the work was recognised when he was awarded the Nobel prize for medicine in 1913. True to tradition, Richet was an allergic subject himself. He could not eat eggs.

As well as establishing the principle of anaphylaxis, Richet established a rule which applies to all allergies from the mildest hay fever to the life-threatening crisis. This is the feature of primary response or 'sensitisation' of the immune system to an allergen. Symptoms are absent when the allergen is encountered for the first time, but they occur when the same antigen is encountered on later occasions, varying in severity according to the individual.

A famous contemporary of Richet, Baron Clemens von Pirquet, was the man who gave the word 'allergy' to the language. Von Pirquet encountered the altered response he named allergy while working as a paediatrician in Vienna. He was well acquainted with immunisation against diphtheria but became seriously concerned to find that a few children were violently ill after injections of diphtheria antitoxin. Some of the sick children died within a short space of time. The violence of their reaction resembled the unexpected death of Richet's dog Neptune. Von Pirquet postulated that the first injection of antitoxin had brought about an altered reactive state in these children and to describe it he coined the word 'allergy'. He recognised that an altered response could be beneficial as in the case of immunity or harmful as instanced by allergy and its extreme manifestation, anaphylactic shock.

With a colleague, Bela Schick – who later became a prominent New York doctor – von Pirquet published in 1902 a famous paper on serum sickness or anaphylactic disease. It is now known that serum sickness was caused by a hypersensitive reaction of the immune system to protein in the horse serum used for immunisation. Such animal serums are little used today but a severe reaction similar to serum sickness can be produced by a number of drugs, most notably penicillin.

During the first half of this century, advances were made in a number of directions. The importance of mould spores as a source of allergy was identified for the first time – their spores can be present in greater density than pollen. A Canadian doctor, F T Cadham, is believed to have reported the first case of mould allergy in 1924. His patient was a farmer whose attacks of asthma followed exposure to a mould on grain or the dust from infected straw. Some earlier allergens disappeared: one curious example was lycopodium, the spores of a type of moss. This substance was used in the theatre, particularly in France, to simulate rain, by being scattered upon the stage, and also fire because it burned with a brilliant flame yet left no smouldering residue. Certain asthmatics could not attend the opera because of the effect of lycopodium on their breathing.

Several new allergens seemed to spring up. Orris root, once used commonly in face powder, largely disappeared but the rapid development of the chemical industry with its new products like nylon and the expansion of food manufacturing production have undoubtedly contributed to an increased incidence of allergy.

Advances were made in various fields of treatment. One pioneer was a young surgeon, Leonard Noon, who was researching bacteria at St Mary's Hospital, Paddington, in 1911, when he decided to turn his attention to grass pollen. Working with a colleague, John Freeman, he discovered that injections of grass pollen dissolved in water could bring relief to sufferers from hay fever – this was a form of desensitisation. Results were published in *The Lancet* the same year. Noon's successors have helped to establish one of the world's leading allergy clinics at St Mary's.

Another important breakthrough was the discovery that hypersensitivity could be transferred from one person to another in blood. Once again, this advance was demonstrated by doctors who themselves suffered from allergies. Carl Prausnitz (1876–1963) suffered from hay fever while Heinz Küstner (1897–1961) developed urticaria after eating fish. Serum from Küstner was injected into Prausnitz's arm. The following day Prausnitz's arm was tested with fish extract and for the first time in his life produced a positive skin reaction to fish. The 'passive transfer test' came to be known by the names of the two men.

It was not until the 1960s that IgE, the immunoglobulin responsible for allergic reaction, was finally identified. Working in the USA, the husband and wife team Kimishige and Teruko Ishizaka announced their discovery of a new group of antibodies, IgE. In the same decade, two immunologists working in the UK, P G H Gell and R R A Coombs, published a classification of allergic reactions still in use today.

Both pieces of research are fundamental in the understanding of allergy and are covered in detail in the next chapter.

2

What is allergy?

The immune system

Immunology, the study of the body's immune system in sickness and health, has been called the science of the future. Discoveries published one year are soon out of date because new findings have changed the picture in the interval. Immunology is important in virtually every field of research, particularly, for instance, in that of organ transplants: it is the immune system which may reject a transplanted organ.

The immune system is supposed to protect the body against a virus or other invading substance. A **defective** immune system provides fewer defences against infection than it should, whereas a **hypersensitive** one overreacts to certain substances which would not bring about the same response in people with normally functioning immune systems: this is allergy.

One of the immune system's most important functions – certainly the most widely appreciated – is the ability to make antibodies (protective agents) against invading substances called antigens.

When an organism invades the body, the immune system sweeps into action. If disease in the form of infection is involved, the symptoms suffered by the patient are caused by the immune system rather than the bacterium or virus involved. For example, a boil is brought about by a bacterial infection. Yet the pain, inflammation and swelling are not caused by the bacterium but by the response of the immune system in trying to prevent the spread of infection.

When the immune system is defective or becomes impaired, the consequences can be grave. The most serious example is the AIDS virus. AIDS (acquired immune deficiency syndrome) causes a serious impairment of the immune system so that victims often succumb to infection after infection. They frequently die as a result of pneumonia or cancer.

Starvation also seriously damages the immune system's ability to function, the reason for famine victims' vulnerability to infection. An attack of chickenpox in a child suffering from severe malnourishment looks like smallpox and often proves fatal.

As another example, the experiments of Josef Mengele at Auschwitz permanently impaired the immune system in his victims. He repeatedly exposed them to induced infection at the camp and as a result their immune systems broke down, leaving them constantly prone to infection.

So, although allergies can cause untold misery, even death sometimes, allergy sufferers should perhaps not curse their hypersensitive immune systems as much as they do: one that is defective is much more hazardous.

How allergy works

Antibodies
Allergies occur in people who have hypersensitive immune systems prone to malfunction. For them, even if an invading organism is not potentially harmful, the alarm bell sounds and it is 'all systems go' in response to the most harmless substances, such as grains of pollen or food proteins that cause no problems for the majority of people.

Just as antibodies are produced in defence against bacteria and viruses, so a special group of antibodies are involved in allergies. Immunoglobulins (the scientific term for antibodies), all found in blood serum, are divided into five groups.

Immunoglobulin E (IgE) is the antibody responsible for allergic reactions. It is the most recent of the groups to have been identified.

The other four groups are listed here for interest but, apart from IgG, appear not to be directly relevant in an allergic response:

- **IgG** the most abundant antibody, forming 75 per cent of the total serum immunoglobulin level. Active in response to bacteria and viruses, it is also recognised as the 'blocking antibody' capable of preventing IgE from triggering allergic response
- **IgA** only present to a small extent, it is concerned with protection at mucosal surfaces and in the gut: present in tears, sweat and saliva
- **IgM** the largest immunoglobulin, it is the first to appear in immune response but does not persist for long
- **IgD** only present in small quantity: active against food antigens.

Types of allergic reaction
Two British immunologists, P G H Gell and R R A Coombs, published in the 1960s a classification of allergic reactions – this is still in use. New research suggests that the four categories they defined will have to be expanded. However, most immunologists now prefer to use the word 'allergy' only to refer to the immediate Type I hypersensitivity.

- **Type I** immediate or anaphylactic: involving IgE and the subsequent release of powerful chemicals from body cells, this group includes disorders dealt with in this book, for example atopic asthma, hay fever and eczema
- **Type II** includes blood transfusion reactions and many autoimmune diseases (outside the scope of this book)
- **Type III** involving immune 'complexes': includes serum sickness, and possibly rheumatoid arthritis and other adverse reactions to food (see Chapter 8)
- **Type IV** delayed sensitivity: contact dermatitis (see Chapter 3); possibly involved in other allergic reactions, although this is controversial.

Type I An essential role is played by one type of white blood cell, called lymphocytes, in both immune and allergic response. These lymphocytes are divided into T cells which originate in the thymus gland at the base of the neck, and B cells which mature in the bone marrow. They circulate throughout the blood and tissues, functioning for as long as twenty years.

This makes them ideal subjects for development of 'memory', one of two most important qualities of the immune system. The other is their ability to produce many millions of different antibodies, each specific to an individual invading antigen.

In its defence strategy, the immune system operates in two ways:

- The T cells attack invading antigens and activate other cells to take defensive measures (cell-mediated immunity).
- The B cells produce antibodies in the blood (humoral immunity).

It is the second reaction which is involved in allergic response:

- Even before an allergen is encountered for the first time, a small number of B cells are ready to react with it because of the nature of their surfaces.
- When an allergen comes along for the first time, it 'locks into' the specific B cells for which it has an affinity.
- This causes the B cells to divide, some of the progeny becoming plasma cells which secrete and then produce antibodies.
- The IgE level in the blood serum rises.

However, plasma cells only live for a short time so after a few weeks the IgE level drops. This constitutes a **primary response** or **sensitisation** and does not give rise to symptoms because the number of cells involved is small.

Not all the B cells convert into plasma cells to produce antibodies. Some survive as long-living 'memory' cells primed to react with much greater ferocity on later encounters with the same allergen. The primary response results in the multiplication of both B and T cells which ensures

26

that later reactions with the same allergen will produce symptoms varying in severity according to the individual.

Two other body cells which play a key role in allergic reactions are:

- **mast cells,** found in the respiratory and gastro-intestinal tracts and in the skin
- **basophils,** found in the blood.

The IgE antibody is attracted to both these cells. Many thousands may collect on a single cell. Mast cells and basophils both contain tiny packets of chemical granules, each surrounded by its own membrane to keep it separate from the others. When an allergen reacts with a specific IgE antibody on the surface of a mast cell or basophil, it triggers the release of chemicals from the granules inside the cell. This process is called degranulation.

It is the chemicals released by this process which cause the many symptoms of allergy.

A Type I allergic reaction

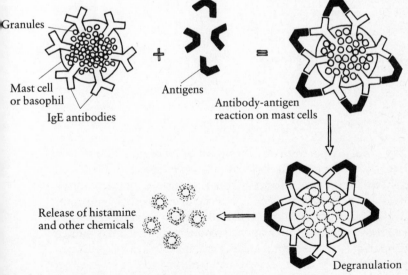

Granules

Mast cell or basophil

IgE antibodies

Antigens

Antibody-antigen reaction on mast cells

Release of histamine and other chemicals

Degranulation

Adapted from a diagram in *Immunology simplified* (OUP 1984)

One of the first of these to be identified was histamine. More recently it has been discovered that the cell membranes of the mast cells and nearby tissue cells release arachidonic acid. This in turn reacts with enzymes to produce chemicals called leukotrienes and prostaglandins. Leukotrienes are known to be thousands of times more powerful than histamine.

The combination of these chemicals produces the three reactions manifested in allergic reactions:

- dilatation of small blood vessels with increased permeability (or leakiness) – the basis for urticaria, angioedema, nasal blockage and allergic headache
- smooth muscle spasm, which produces the contraction of the airways typical of asthma; it is also probably responsible for the spasms which accompany gastro-intestinal allergy
- increased secretions which are evident in allergic conjunctivitis, ear disorders, asthma and hay fever.

It is known that all three chemicals are active in asthma, for instance. Histamine contracts the central bronchial passages, while leukotrienes are mainly responsible for the narrowing of peripheral airways. Prostaglandins, a group of fatty acids, also constrict the air passages.

Reaction to histamine produces the thin watery mucus and provokes the itching and sneezing typical of hay fever.

Fluid leaking from small blood vessels is responsible for the typical weals of urticaria and the swelling of the deeper layers of the skin and underlying tissue which occurs in angioedema (see Chapter 7). White blood cells called eosinophils congregate at the site of an allergic reaction as a result of the degranulation of mast cells.

In its most severe form a Type I reaction is called anaphylactic shock and involves all areas of the body. Symptoms include urticaria all over the body, severe swelling of the tissues including the throat, pain and vomiting and a sudden drop in blood pressure – see Chapter 9.

Type II reaction is outside the scope of this book.

Type III In this type of allergic reaction, immune complexes circulating in the blood are formed by a combination of antibodies and allergens. They are usually eliminated by the immune system and cause only transient symptoms.

Occasionally – depending on a number of factors, including their site and size – they persist, causing acute or chronic symptoms. Serum sickness (see Chapter 10) and farmers' lung (see Chapter 5) are examples. One current theory is that this reaction may be involved in delayed symptoms to food (see Chapter 8). Chapter 8 also gives a fuller explanation of the nature of Type III immune complexes.

Type IV Unlike a Type I reaction, this is a cell-mediated immune response (see page 26). It includes both transplant rejection and contact eczema and is a delayed type of reaction. In eczema, the allergens are called haptens – typical examples are hormones or other drugs. Haptens combine with protein in the skin to form a complete allergen – in other words it can act as an allergen by itself on future occasions. More on the nature of this reaction can be found in Chapter 3 under Contact dermatitis.

Incidence of allergy

Incidence of allergy has been put as high as 50 per cent of the population in developed countries, although there is a remarkable dearth of statistics to support the case that allergies are increasing all the time. The World Health Organisation, however, perceives an increase in the incidence of allergy, particularly in developing countries.

There are two main reasons for this perceived increase. Firstly, allergic conditions are more often correctly diagnosed than they were in the past. Secondly, the proliferation of man-made substances – in the form of pesticides, food additives, pharmaceuticals and synthetic materials like nylon and plastic – has multiplied the potential sources of allergy. A further contributory factor could be a reduction in the practice of breast-feeding in some countries.

It is generally appreciated that the itch of eczema, the sneezing of hay fever and the wheezing of asthma may be due to allergies. However, there is a growing school of thought which believes that food allergy in particular may be responsible for a much wider range of symptoms, from depression and headaches to arthritis and even alcoholism in some people.

Some of the doctors who take this view describe themselves as clinical ecologists or – a more recent term – practitioners of environmental medicine. On the other hand, a number of distinguished allergists at leading hospitals have conducted studies which break new ground. Some of their results are given in this book.

This new approach to food allergy (see Chapter 8) suggests that there are many more sufferers than used to be thought and that allergy has outstripped infection as the major cause of disease.

In terms of demands on medical resources and the cause of disability, conventional allergies rank among the top three to six diseases in developed countries, according to WHO. In developing countries the resources are not available to diagnose and treat atopic illness and the field has been neglected. WHO warns that a number of these countries are fast reaching the stage where appropriate care for allergic patients will have to be tackled.

Illustration *This instance showing how increasing affluence can introduce allergies to a country for the first time was given in* Clinical Allergy *(journal of the British Society for Allergy and Clinical Immunology). A detailed survey in Kuwait was published in 1984 reporting that before the mid-1950s allergy was not considered a problem there. Situated on the north-west shores of the Persian Gulf, Kuwait had hot, dry summers and mild winters. Sandstorms occurred regularly, most frequently in summer.*

More recently allergy had developed to such an extent that 18 per cent of Kuwait's population was estimated to suffer from some type of atopic disorder. A study of 1,000 asthmatic patients attending a central clinic was made over a three-year period.

The principal allergen responsible for most positive skin tests was pollen, mainly from the mesquite tree which was imported from Iran in 1951 and planted in very large numbers when water became available. The chief pollinating seasons were March– April and September–November. The greatest number of asthmatics came to the clinic between April and October. Kuwait had halted the planting of mesquite trees but the damage had been done: they were already there in abundance.

Many patients had associated conditions: 63 per cent hay fever, 35 per cent conjunctivitis and 27 per cent urticaria and/or angioedema. Few people kept pets and this was reflected in a low incidence of hypersensitivity to animals. The research team was surprised to find that reactions to the house-dust mite were also rare. A possible explanation was that although the temperatures in Kuwait were suitable for the mite, the comparatively low humidity was not. For the same reason, moulds were not prevalent.

Forty-seven per cent of the patients had close members of the family suffering from allergies but among the Bedouins the figure increased to 64 per cent. The reason suggested was that inter-marriage was greater in this group than among Kuwaiti town dwellers.

What happened in Kuwait is being duplicated in countries all over the world, with variations according to many different circumstances. This led to a special conference called by the World Health Organisation in Florence in 1984 to discuss the avoidance of allergens; a report is in preparation, due for publication in 1986.

Statistics

Statistics relating to allergy must be regarded with caution. Research often produces widely differing statistical results in the course of similar projects. One example was quoted at a WHO conference held in Geneva in 1978. In one study, 29,996 medical students were interviewed and an incidence of allergy of 12.49 per cent was estimated. In a second investigation of 10,413 subjects – also medical students – the percentage suffering from allergic disorders was 6.38.

Some of the other reasons for variations in statistics concerning allergy are that:

- allergic diseases are not defined in a uniform fashion. In general, only Type I reactions are included
- no absolute criteria are set down for interpreting the results of allergy tests
- diagnosis, particularly in developing countries, may be deficient because medical teams lack training in the field of allergy
- patients with mild allergies may sometimes be excluded from results
- selection of subjects may introduce bias
- many studies are based on information supplied subjectively by the patients, not on positive controlled immune tests.

Other aspects of allergy

While it is true that allergies are increasing, it is also the case that life is now much safer and more comfortable for sufferers, particularly in developed countries.

It is widely known that allergies run in families. However, it is not a specific condition which is inherited but a general atopic tendency. Not all members of a family are affected to the same degree: some may escape altogether apart from an isolated incident or two.

It is less widely known that the date of birth may contribute to the development of allergies. In his paper in the WHO report on allergies to be published in 1986, Professor Jack Pepys observes that infants under six months old seem to be the most susceptible to pollen allergy, and that in the UK birth between May and October is associated with house-dust mite allergy and between December and February with grass pollens.

The report also makes it clear that although race and heredity undoubtedly feature in allergy, they are less important than environmental influences in early childhood, in the development of asthma, for example. Studies have shown that children living in the UK who were born in the West Indies, Africa, India and Pakistan tend to develop allergies less than immigrant children born in the UK, who fall in with the pattern of all children in the UK.

What makes allergy worse

Allergic or allergic-like symptoms can be exacerbated by a number of different factors including:

- **infection** many young children wheeze for the first time with a bad cold and the presence of infection can seriously complicate infantile eczema; severe infection of the gut may encourage the development of allergy
- **emotional disturbance** it is possible for fear or distress to trigger an asthmatic attack
- **weather** bright, windy weather can carry pollens con- siderable distances while mild, damp weather increases the incidence of spores.

Tolerance level

There may also sometimes be a question of degree. Sensi- tivity to a particular food, for example, is not absolute. Many patients have a 'tolerance level' so that someone allergic to wheat may be able to eat one slice of bread daily without symptoms, but more will provoke a reaction. If the sufferer is also pollen-sensitive, he may not be able to eat his one slice of bread without symptoms during the pollen season.

In other people, only minute quantities of an allergen are necessary to produce reactions. Even the smell of coffee or fish, for example, is enough to bring on symptoms in hypersensitive people.

Pseudoallergy

There is also the phenomenon of 'pseudoallergy'. Its fun- damental difference from true allergic reaction can be appreciated by repeating the sequence of events involving

IgE antibodies. A specific allergen reacts with IgE antibodies produced as a result of an earlier (sensitising) encounter with the same substance. The ultimate effect is the release of chemicals from mast cells and basophils which cause the symptoms of allergy according to their site in the body.

Pseudoallergy is triggered – in many instances – by a chemical compound which has the ability to react *directly* with mast cells, stimulating them to release histamine. This type of reaction also differs from true allergy in that symptoms can occur when the substance is encountered for the first time. The early sensitisation, which is an invariable feature of hypersensitivity, does not apply. Initial reactions can sometimes be violent.

Diagnosis

If you suspect you are suffering from a serious allergic reaction, ask your doctor's advice. Many GPs who are not specialists in the field will refer patients to an allergy clinic.

You should be ready to answer a wide range of questions about your day-to-day life. Any of the following methods may be used to identify the cause of your allergy.

Case histories
All investigations of allergy begin with a detailed case history. When you first go to an allergy clinic, say, the relevance of some of the information required will not always be obvious to you. However, a painstaking picture of your way of life, built up month after month, will provide valuable clues to diagnosis.

Even so, tracing the cause of an individual allergy is still far from straightforward. For example, there may be a number of contributing allergens, some inhaled and others eaten. You may consult a doctor about an isolated symptom but careful questioning may eventually reveal a much more complicated picture.

Case history *A 35-year-old female patient consulted an allergist, complaining of nasal congestion. However, investigation re-*

vealed other longstanding symptoms – headache, constipation and abdominal pain. Tests and treatment proved that the gastro-intestinal symptoms were caused by cow's milk. She was also found to be allergic to inhaled moulds, pollens and cat dander, and these were the principal causes of her nasal congestion. However, milk was shown to contribute to the nasal symptoms and it also proved responsible for her headaches.

Clinics use charts – either provided by the company market-ing the allergen samples or designed by the hospital – for patients to take home and fill in over a specified period. Housing, occupation, hobbies, holidays, family relationships, emotional ups and downs and diet are all relevant in a case history. You also have to give details of your symptoms with an indication of severity on a daily basis.

It may be necessary to keep a chart over several months. If symptoms persist all the year round, it is likely that the cause can be traced to the dust mite – or just the family pet. (Sometimes a family finds it difficult to believe that a much-loved animal is the source of a child's illness. One doctor on an emergency call to a child suffering an acute attack of asthma noticed a budgerigar acquired since his last visit. He did not succeed in convincing the parents that the removal of the bird would probably cure the child and they still urged him to admit her to hospital. He explained that this too was likely to cure the asthma – because the child would have been taken away from the bird.)

Skin tests

The case history may well indicate which skin tests are likely to prove positive but a standard range will normally be performed. These tests have a long history and are widely recognised as the principal method for tracing substances responsible for allergic symptoms. Two methods used are:

- a prick test using a sterile lancet or needle; one drop of each test solution is used

- **an intradermal test** which involves injecting a higher dose of allergen under the skin. There is therefore a greater risk of anaphylactic shock (see Chapter 9). Although it is commonly used in the USA, it is employed in the UK only rarely, when the prick test is negative.

Skin tests are most reliable in confirming allergy to inhaled substances but they are also useful when hypersensitivity to a food, an insect or an anaesthetic is suspected. Some allergists are sceptical about results because often they do not correlate with a patient's symptoms: positive reactions can be produced in individuals who do not suffer from any atopic disorder.

However, skin testing remains a first-line diagnostic tool, cheap, safe and easy to perform, and often corroborating allergens already under suspicion from a case history. A positive weal and flare reaction occurs within minutes of a test. It is important that the tests are carried out precisely by trained staff.

Challenge or provocation test

This form of test has the same basic concept as skin tests although it is performed in different ways according to the type of disorder. Conjunctival challenge, which involves introducing a drop of allergen into the eye, is seldom used because of the risk involved (see Chapter 4).

The two tests most frequently performed are nasal and bronchial challenge.

In **nasal challenge**, the allergen can be administered:

- in powdered form by spray
- in solution from a bottle dropper or syringe
- by application on a cottonbud.

It is important that patients hold their breath and exhale 30 seconds later to prevent the allergen reaching the lower airways where it could provoke asthma in sensitive individuals. The results can be assessed by:

- counting sneezes in the following 15 minutes
- measuring nasal discharge
- examining the inside of the nose.

The role of **bronchial challenge** is controversial, although it is useful in instances where diagnosis is difficult or other tests have failed to identify the allergen. In one study, 30 per cent of patients with negative skin tests to house dust produced positive results to bronchial provocation.

A number of sophisticated techniques are employed. The most common is performed with a nebuliser. A seated patient breathes in a measured quantity of the chosen agent; a spirometer then measures forced expiratory flow in one second. It is important that the patient breathes deeply so that the substance is taken into the lungs. The most common agent used in solution in a nebuliser is histamine but sometimes it is a suspected allergen or even methacholine, a chemical to which asthmatics are highly sensitive. Occasionally, hospitals specialising in the treatment of industrial asthma have test rooms which simulate conditions in the patient's place of work.

There is a risk of severe anaphylaxis in a very small number of patients and in the case of bronchial challenge the subject is normally kept in hospital for at least 48 hours because delayed responses sometimes occur.

However, information can be obtained from strictly conducted tests of this kind which is not available by other methods.

Laboratory tests
In addition to these tests allergists can now obtain back-up from a range of laboratory tests. The simplest is to **look for eosinophils** – white blood cells always present at the site of an allergic reaction. This is usually done by taking samples of sputum and secretions from nose and eye – all of which provide more reliable results than blood samples. Eosinophils are easily recognised dye-stained under the microscope.

In the majority of people the level of IgE antibody present in blood serum is low. It has been found to be 100 times the normal level in some atopic individuals. However, measurable IgE does not provide infallible corroboration of allergy because it can be mildly elevated in people who are free of symptoms. This is just one aspect of hypersensitivity which is still poorly understood.

However, there now exists a test which is much more useful than the measurement of total IgE. **RAST** (radioallergosorbent) **assays** can measure specific IgE – that is, specific to an individual allergen. The development of this test marked a major advance in the diagnosis of allergy. However, as it is a very expensive procedure, many allergists still regard skin testing as the prime tool of diagnosis.

Methods of treatment

Methods of treatment are also covered in the chapters on particular allergies. An immense variety of drugs is available for the treatment of allergies. Some of the more widely used ones are described here.

Steroids

Steroids used in the treatment of allergy, particularly for eczema and asthma, are laboratory-produced hormones similar to the cortisone produced by the body. They are more correctly called corticosteroids because in the body they originate in the cortex, part of the adrenal glands which are situated just above the kidneys. What makes them so important in the field of allergy is their powerful ability to suppress allergic inflammation.

Individual corticosteroids were identified in the 1930s, including cortisone and the closely related hydrocortisone. The production of these hormones by the adrenal cortex was discovered to be governed by yet another hormone, ACTH, which is secreted by the pituitary, a tiny gland situated at the base of the brain.

In the 1940s scientists came to suggest that stress affecting the brain increased production of ACTH from the pituitary which – in turn – increased the production of cortico-steroids. It was known that during pregnancy – when the production of hormones soars – patients with arthritis experienced a reduction in pain. When other arthritic patients were treated with cortisone, they too improved dramatically.

Steroids, as they are generally known today, began to be used for a very wide range of diseases, including asthma. At first, results seemed almost magical for many patients. The powerful ability to dampen down inflammation with its attendant distress made the new discovery look like a major breakthrough for medicine.

However, it was soon discovered that their continual use in high doses could result in a list of formidable side effects. Their use waned as patients' anxiety increased and doctors began to appreciate that these were drugs to be used with great discretion and that high dosage treatment for a short time was only justified by severe conditions which did not respond to other treatment.

Over the years, several possible side effects have come to be associated with treatment by steroids:

- stunting of growth – this can only occur when relatively high doses are required to control severe eczema or asthma (principally with systemic treatment, ie given by injection or mouth)
- swelling of the face, known as 'moonface', which only occurs when a great deal of oral steroid has been absorbed into the bloodstream
- eye problems including cataracts which can cause loss of vision – these only result from systemic therapy
- adrenal suppression – the body loses its natural ability to produce steroids in conditions of stress, for example in cases of accident (this only occurs when treatment is systemic)
- a stretching and thinning of the skin known as 'atrophy', especially when a strong steroid has been applied topically.

This is not a complete list of side effects that have been claimed for steroid treatment, but it is sufficiently alarming to disturb particularly parents of an allergic child.

Steroids are available in different forms: in creams and ointments of varying strengths for the treatment of eczema and in inhalers for asthmatics and hayfever patients. Side effects are now much less of a problem than they used to be because fewer steroid preparations are taken by mouth. However, tablets are still prescribed for particularly serious conditions, very often for a short period to deal with a crisis or for longer periods to control a serious condition. In this instance it is most important that patients should wear a Medic-Alert bracelet or pendant giving information about the treatment (the address is given at the back of the book); or they can ask their doctor for a steroid card.

A problem occurs because if systemic treatment has been in progress for one month or more, the cortex progressively loses its ability to increase its production of corticosteroids in response to stress. If the patient encounters a stressful situation – an accident, for example – failure to increase production of steroids can lead to collapse or even death. An increased dose of corticosteroids can save a patient's life in this situation so the information about treatment must be available to the medical help summoned to the accident.

Adrenaline

The inner part of the adrenal gland, the medulla, also has a link with modern treatment for allergy. The hormones it produces are adrenaline and noradrenaline (epinephrine and norepinephrine in the USA). In face of danger, these hormones are pumped into the bloodstream. The activity of the heart is stepped up, providing more blood for the brain and muscles. Breathing becomes faster and deeper, drawing in more oxygen. Increased perspiration cools the body. Muscles tighten in preparation for vigorous action and the pupils dilate, making the eyes more sensitive.

Adrenaline, like corticosteroids, can now be synthesised in the laboratory. Its powerful stimulatory effect makes it the standard international treatment for the most severe symptom of allergy – anaphylaxis (see Chapter 9). A pre-filled syringe is available in the UK and a doctor may recommend that a patient at serious risk keep an emergency kit of this kind available.

Sodium cromoglycate (SCG)

Another drug of importance in the field of allergy is sodium cromoglycate (SCG), which has negligible side effects. It does not work by reducing inflammation, nor does it have the effect of drugs known as bronchodilators, which open up the narrowed airways of the lungs during an attack of asthma (see Chapter 5). Its effect is believed to be directly on mast cells, preventing the release of chemicals responsible for symptoms of allergy (see earlier in the chapter). Its use has recently been extended from the fields of eyes and nasal and bronchial allergy to treat food allergies. However, there are some allergists who believe that the value of SCG is exaggerated in food allergy problems.

Antihistamines

Antihistamines, well known as a treatment for hay fever, are also used in the treatment of many other allergic conditions. They can be given by mouth or as an injection for an allergic emergency. They work by blocking the effects of histamine, which is one of the chemicals produced in the mast cells in an allergic reaction.

Immunotherapy

Immunotherapy, also known as desensitisation or hypo-sensitisation, is sometimes an effective treatment for asthma and hay fever (see Chapters 5 and 6), and more frequently for allergy to insect stings (Chapter 9).

In 1911 when Leonard Noon and John Freeman announced that the very grass extracts that brought on hay fever, when dissolved in water, could be used to reduce the symptoms of sufferers from hay fever, there were great hopes that this type of therapy would hold the answer for all sufferers from allergy. Unfortunately, this did not prove to be so although immunotherapy is used extensively for inhalant allergies in the USA, Europe and elsewhere in the world, and to a much lesser extent in the UK.

The premise on which Noon and Freeman based their hopes was a mistaken one. They believed that a toxin was produced in the body by the inhalation of grass pollens and so their method was an extension of standard immunisation against disease. By injecting small quantities of pollens over a period, immunity to their effect would be built up in the sensitive patient.

Since the discovery of IgE antibodies and the mechanism of allergic reaction as a malfunction of the immune system, this assumption has been disproved. Modern allergists cannot explain exactly how immunotherapy works. There is even some controversy as to whether it does work although there is a consensus that it is effective for some people and less so for others. Allergists in the UK tend to regard immunotherapy as a last-ditch measure when drug treatment has proved ineffective.

It is now believed that the principal effect of the therapy is to stimulate the production of IgG antibodies, sometimes called 'the blocking antibody', in other words the antibody capable of preventing the production of IgE which leads to allergic symptoms. No trials carried out have yet produced clear evidence of this.

Immunotherapy studies have been carried out with ragweed hay fever subjects in the USA which have shown that while IgE specific to ragweed increased in untreated patients during the pollination season, after initial increase it began to fall in those receiving treatment. At the end of one two-year study, 18 out of 19 treated patients had decreased levels of IgE specific to ragweed.

Research

Despite great advances in the field of allergy, enabling acute attacks to be contained and chronic symptoms alleviated, many general practitioners still fail to appreciate the importance of allergy as a factor to be considered in a wide spectrum of disease. No-one could expect family doctors to keep abreast of the rapid advances in allergy and immunology: all specialist fields are becoming too vast for the general physician to maintain up-to-date knowledge of any of them. Even so, too often general practitioners fail to refer a patient to an allergy clinic when such a referral might well be of great benefit. Equally, some specialists are sceptical of the work done by allergists. For example, many dermatologists are unconvinced of the role played by diet in atopic eczema. Many controversies and anomalies complicate a picture which is already vastly complex.

However, research is taking place in many countries and although it may still be impossible to effect a total cure for any condition, the next decade is likely to witness great improvements in treatments (see Postscript). Perhaps the most important areas of research, because they are likely to have the most wide-reaching implications, are those into Type III immune complexes, and into the role played by antibodies other than IgE.

3

Eczema

Any skin ailment is distressing but a baby suffering from eczema is a uniquely pitiful sight. It is natural that parents should be disturbed even if the disfiguring condition is comparatively mild and responds well to the wide variety of treatments now available. However, severe eczema in a young baby can disrupt the life of an entire family and cause parents terrible anxiety.

What is eczema?

Symptoms
Eczema is typically a disorder of infancy, but it can persist into childhood and beyond. Its first appearance is often on the baby's face, progressing later to the trunk, arms and legs. Typically, it settles in the creases inside the arms and at the back of the legs. Wrists and ankles also seem vulnerable. Its first appearance might be no more than a slight red rash that parents would dismiss as trivial and transitory. However, eczema has one outstanding symptom which can never be ignored and is the main cause of the misery it produces. It is undoubtedly the itchiest skin condition which afflicts mankind.

Every baby with eczema scratches, often more at night. The irritation is so severe and invariable that some doctors in the past believed that the rash was caused by the scratching rather than the other way round.

Increased redness of the skin is the earliest symptom of worsening eczema. One of the classic symptoms of any allergy is extra leakiness of the blood vessels, allowing fluid to seep out. In eczema this has the effect of forming small fluid-filled blisters called 'vesicles' which weep and even bleed when broken by scratching, and then form crusts because of the presence of clotting agents in the blood.

All eczema sufferers tend to have dry scaly skin. As the child grows older, continual scratching causes the skin to become thickened and leathery and the normal skin lines become exaggerated. This condition can persist and remain itchy long after the original rash has cleared up. Some individuals have the condition known as 'ichthyosis' (from Greek 'ikhthus': fish), so named because the skin comes to resemble fish scales.

A child with severe eczema is vulnerable to complicating skin infections. These do not occur frequently but one condition is potentially serious. The herpes virus can be responsible for a superimposed rash, resembling the blistering of eczema, which can be dangerous. For this reason, no-one with a cold sore on their lips – caused by the herpes virus – should have any physical contact with a child suffering from eczema. If it is another member of the family who is affected, the cold sore must be covered with a dressing.

If there is a sudden worsening of an eczema condition with increased blistering, and the child seems unwell and feverish, medical help is needed without delay.

In rare cases, the virus can reach internal organs from the infected skin. A drug is available (which must be given intravenously) which prevents the viral infection spreading. This is Zovirax (acyclovir – the Wellcome Foundation received a Queen's Award for technical achievement in 1985 for its discovery). The drug is believed to be the first safe and effective treatment for the herpes virus.

Bacterial and fungal infections of the skin are fairly common in conjunction with eczema and these may be less obvious than the more serious viral infection. Nevertheless, they do make the condition worse and a swab may need to be taken in hospital to identify the infection and treat it.

Occasionally, a child has to be admitted to hospital. This should not be regarded as failure where severe eczema is concerned. Invariably, there is a considerable improvement in the child's condition and it does provide a much needed break for other members of the family.

Sufferers

One specialist, Dr David Atherton, Consultant Dermatologist at London's Hospital for Sick Children, Great Ormond Street, judges that if a child has eczema at the age of one year, there is a better than 50:50 chance that it will no longer be a problem by the time he is five; of the remaining children still affected then, only about 20 per cent will have troublesome eczema at the age of 10 and only 5 per cent by the age of 15.

In general, the later it develops the more intractable it proves. Often, it seems to be the rash which develops with some severity around the age of ten (perhaps after mild outbreaks in earlier years) which proves most persistent. Sometimes the eczema clears up in adolescence.

Many women find that their skin condition improves dramatically during pregnancy. This is a reaction observed in a wide variety of chronic ailments, many of them unrelated to allergy, and is generally believed to be due to the hormonal changes taking place.

However, as in all allergies, eczema is a highly individualised disorder and although a general pattern is discernible, many people do not conform to it. A small minority suffer from eczema all their lives and for an unlucky few the symptoms remain severe.

Types of eczema

Dermatologists recognise many different types of eczema, but a basic division into three categories is useful when the allergic factor is the main consideration:

- **atopic eczema** where there is a tendency to inherit the skin condition, and where there is a reaction to allergens – these may be eaten or drunk (such as eggs or milk) or inhaled (such as pollen or dust mites). It is particularly common in infancy
- **contact eczema** (often called dermatitis) which is a delayed Type IV allergic reaction (see Chapter 2) so may take months or even years to develop; sometimes it appears after the person starts work when the contact allergen is encountered for the first time. People with atopic eczema, an inborn condition, are thought by some allergists to be less likely to develop contact eczema than non-atopics
- **irritant eczema** which can be caused by everyday substances such as washing powder and detergents. Having a dry flaky skin, the atopic individual is particularly vulnerable, so this type of eczema may become obvious in babyhood.

(Two terms also used in reference to eczema are endogenous – an inherited atopic form – and exogenous – a contact reaction to an outside agent.)

Atopic eczema

Preventive measures

Despite the general conviction that allergies are becoming more widespread – some estimates gauge that 30 per cent of the population are atopic – there are few reliable statistics to support the view. One useful exception is a study, reported in the British Medical Journal (BMJ) in September 1983, indicating that atopic eczema is 'rising alarmingly'. In an investigation of 12,555 children born in a single week in 1970, it was discovered that 12.3 per cent developed eczema by the age of five. This was more than twice the proportion affected in a similar study 12 years earlier.

A baby's chances of developing eczema depend – to a great extent – upon heredity. A recent Swedish study produced the following results:

- where there was no history of parental allergies, six per cent of children under the age of seven developed atopic eczema
- when one parent had such a history, the figure doubled to 12 per cent
- if both parents were affected, the figure rose to 33 per cent.

Medical opinion is unanimous that breast-feeding is best for all babies, but it is particularly beneficial for those at risk from allergies (because one or both parents suffer from atopic reactions of some nature). The BMJ article in 1983 (by Dr Atherton – see above) concluded that exclusive breast-feeding for at least 12 weeks provided some protection for infants at risk.

This is because human milk contains IgA as well as a factor which accelerates further production of this protective antibody. The WHO report on Prevention of Allergies (1986) refers to studies of babies born to atopic parents in which those who developed infantile eczema showed lower IgA levels than those who did not.

It is also generally believed that breast-feeding – as well as helping prevent eczema in babyhood – provides some defence against allergies in later life.

However, it does not give complete protection because breast-fed babies occasionally do develop eczema. One theory is that an atopic mother may transmit food allergens to the baby in her milk. If she knows that she is herself even slightly allergic to cow's milk, it would be wise to avoid it altogether while she is breast-feeding. Milk contains essential calcium (not easily replaced by diet) and if she is going to avoid it entirely, she should take calcium tablets to supply the missing element (as well as extra protein).

In some hospitals it is still quite common to give a newly born baby a supplementary feed based on cow's milk in order to let a mother have an undisturbed night's sleep. The best obstetric units have now abandoned this practice because of general acceptance that cow's milk – even in small quantities – can sensitise an infant and increase the risk of eczema. A mother who knows that her baby is at risk because there is a family history of allergies should alert the staff at her maternity unit if her doctor has not raised the matter first. Even if breast-feeding is going well, the only supplement given to the baby should be dextrose solution (a form of glucose).

However, if breast-feeding is medically impossible, there are a number of alternatives on the market, including soya-based milks, for a baby at risk. These include Prosobee and Nutramigen (both from Mead Johnson), Wysoy (Wyeth), and Formula S (Cow & Gate). Pregestimil (a 'pre-digested' cow's milk) may also be prescribed by a consultant for high-risk babies over three months old.

Even if all possible preventive measures are taken, some infants still develop eczema. In some cases parents may not even be aware that there is a family history of atopic illness. Older people often forget the mild allergies of childhood. Sometimes the illnesses skip a generation and cease to be part of family history.

Care and treatment

'Holistic medicine' is one of several therapies covered in Chapter 11. Its precept is that the patient's symptoms can be tackled by treating the whole person, instead of the more conventional approach of considering a set of symptoms and then prescribing medication designed to deal with them alone.

In caring for a child with eczema, especially in cases where the condition is severe, the entire day-to-day life of the child must be governed by an understanding of the many factors involved, from inhaled allergens frequently present in the air to the washing powder used for the child's nappies and the diet from babyhood onwards. Climate and emotional ups and downs, the happy occasions as well as the sad, can all affect the skin.

For many parents there are desperate times: severe eczema is disfiguring and involves trauma to a varying degree for both the sufferer and the family. But there is one overriding comfort for all – however severe, eczema does clear up completely, leaving an unscarred skin and no lasting psychological damage.

Like all allergies, eczema waxes and wanes without discernible reason. Treatment varies from doctor to doctor and no two patients are alike. Very often family doctors have neither the time nor the expert knowledge to give the best guidance. It is important to obtain the best possible advice and this should be by referral to a paediatrician or dermatologist at a local hospital. London's teaching hospitals and many of the leading provincial hospitals have allergy clinics.

Home environment
Even mild eczema in a baby should make parents look about them for factors liable to affect the skin condition – often attended by other allergies – of a growing child. Skin prick tests will reveal the principal allergens and if one of these is the house-dust mite (see Chapter 5) or one of the many other components of dust such as animal dander, simple steps can be taken to reduce the problem.

Parting with a family pet may be difficult but is necessary if its presence is exacerbating a child's condition. A family prone to allergy would be wise to avoid acquiring any pets in the first place because at least one member of the household may be affected.

Furnishings, particularly in the child's bedroom, should be as simple and easy to keep clean as possible – easily washable curtains and rugs rather than fitted carpets and heavy fabrics. Dusting should always be done with a damp cloth, and a vacuum cleaner is preferable to a broom. The child should not be in the room while cleaning is taking place because of the dust disturbed.

Pillows and duvets filled with feathers or down should be

avoided. Mattresses and pillows can be enclosed in plastic covers but taken out regularly for airing and the pillows washed as frequently as possible. Many atopics travel with their own pillows to try to avoid problems away from home.

Clothing

Both wool and nylon are possible irritants so cotton is the best choice for a baby with eczema. The address of Cotton On, a company specialising in the manufacture of cotton clothing for adults and children, can be found at the end of the book. Cotton blankets are also available. It is not sufficient to line a woollen garment with cotton because the wrist is a particularly vulnerable part of the body and the merest contact with wool is often enough to produce a rash. Cotton pyjamas and jumpers with attached mittens, widely used in hospitals, are particularly useful.

Prevention of scratching

Before the development of modern treatment, many babies with severe eczema spent weeks in hospital, well sedated and swaddled in heavy bandages. Bandaging may still be necessary, but the modern alternatives are lightweight, convenient and just as effective. A wide range of cotton tubular bandage is available in sizes (for different age groups) to fit the trunk, limbs and even individual fingers. Mittens to prevent night-time scratching can be improvised easily from this bandage. During the day, a child's hands should if possible be left free; nails must therefore be kept short and gently filed smooth.

A variation is the medicated bandage impregnated with one of a number of different pastes so that the inflamed skin is soothed and scratching prevented at the same time. Coal tar preparations are quite often used (Tarband or Coltapaste) but alternatives may be prescribed.

Avoiding irritants

Although the diagnosis may be atopic eczema, irritant factors from many different sources can worsen the

51

condition (see later in the chapter). The washing powder used for a child's laundry is often found to affect the skin. The introduction of biological washing powders in the early 1980s greatly increased reactions but after representations from the National Eczema Society one of the major companies, Lever Brothers, reintroduced their original 'non-biological' Persil washing powder. Other suitable washing powders are available on a limited scale: the National Eczema Society will supply a list of soap-based products and detergents.

Dressing a child with eczema is sometimes a problem because over-heating, whether from too many clothes, excessive room heating or bath water which is too hot, has a harmful effect on the skin. Direct heat from the sun or an open fire may also irritate although many children benefit from a seaside holiday. (Apparent contradictions such as this commonly occur in the field of allergy where the responses of the individual must always be the final arbiter.)

Eczema sufferers whose hands are affected should always wear gloves – cotton 'liners' inside roomy rubber gloves are a good protection against many detergents and house-cleaning products. For the same reason, neither hairdressing nor nursing is a sensible choice of career; other unsuitable occupations include jobs where contact with dirt and grease means that the hands have to be washed frequently.

Bathing

A child with broken, inflamed and sometimes infected skin will inevitably hate bath-time; it used to be normal practice to avoid bathing a child with eczema altogether. Now, however, there is a choice of products to add to the bath water which soothe and moisturise. As many soaps also have a damaging effect, this moisturiser can be used in their place and the child should take a small pot to school for hand-washing. Bubble-bath should never be added to bath water. Instead, emulsifying ointment (a type of moisturiser) is best used by dissolving two dessertspoonfuls in a jug of boiling water, whisking the mixture with a fork and then adding to the bath so there is an even distribution. As an alternative, small amounts can be dabbed all over the body and stroked gently in one direction.

Claims are made for the curative properties of mineral salts from the Dead Sea. These powers were known in biblical times. King David, King Solomon and the Queen of Sheba built curative bathing palaces on its shores, the forerunners of the spas there today. Dead Sea salt, as well as creams and lotions, is available from some health food shops and by mail order (the address can be found under 'Dead Sea' in the list at the back of the book).

Diet

Skin tests on children with eczema often prove positive to foods that are commonly allergenic, such as milk and eggs. However, these results cannot be seen as infallible proof that the cause of the condition has been found. Because the severity of the rash can vary from day to day, even from hour to hour, it is difficult to prove a link between food and the condition, and some specialists remain sceptical.

In practice, a restricted diet often improves the skin and several studies have shown that two out of three children with eczema benefit when certain foods are cut out. Some dermatologists feel that for mild cases of eczema no restriction is necessary. In more serious cases, milk and eggs, and chicken because some of its proteins are identical to those of eggs, are the first items a dietitian eliminates, being replaced by alternative foods to supply essential nutrients.

If a milk- and egg-free diet is going to help, the improvement will be seen in six weeks or so. It is generally recommended then that the diet be maintained for one year and the foods then re-introduced one at a time in small quantities to see whether they can be tolerated.

Weaning a baby who has eczema needs to be done with care. If cow's milk and eggs have been eliminated, the former should not be given, and then only cautiously in small quantities, until twelve months, and the latter not until eighteen months.

Introduction of solids is best delayed until the child is four months old. One teaspoonful of cereal mixed smoothly with breast milk until it is semi-liquid is a good first choice. In case of adverse reaction, it is sensible to introduce one cereal for a period of a week or two before making a change. In the same way, fruits and vegetables in the form of a purée should be introduced singly. Reaction to food may be either almost immediate or else delayed, so it is safest to establish each new item in the baby's diet to ensure that it can be given safely.

A young child with severe eczema is hardly a subject for experimentation, however well intentioned, but older people sometimes find the most unexpected treatments bring about relief, such as the application of yoghurt or honey to the skin. Other foods often found to be allergenic include nuts, tomatoes, fish, food colourings and preservatives. One woman pinpointed the cause of her own eczema after a period of trial and error as the yellow food colouring, tartrazine (E102).

More information about food allergy can be found in Chapter 8.

Emotion

An unsightly rash is likely to be an emotional problem for a child, particularly when starting school, so it is crucial for parents to explain that eczema is not infectious, and to have a word with the teacher in charge so that any teasing can be nipped in the bud.

Stress has a powerful effect upon all skin disorders and it is important for anyone with atopic eczema to bear this in mind when choosing a career.

Steroids

Details are given in Chapter 2 about the nature and history of steroids.

Laboratory-produced steroids have a powerful anti-inflammatory action. Used in the form of creams and ointments, they are described as 'topical' because they are applied to the site of the inflammation (from Greek 'topos': place). If given by injection or mouth to reach body organs through the blood, they are called 'systemic' steroids.

While it is true that steroids can give rise to considerable side effects, particularly if taken systemically, they can be extremely helpful in the management of eczema. Many people using the latest forms of topical steroids experience no side effects. Of those who do, the most common side effect is the thinning of the skin. A typical instance is a woman of 34 who in her teens was prescribed a steroid cream of medium potency which she used on her face every two days for about ten years. As a result she felt that she looked ten years older than she was because her skin was very thin and lined.

However, in the comparatively rare cases where a strong steroid ointment is required to control severe eczema, it is dangerous to discontinue treatment. For example, one mother took her child off steroid preparations for a whole year after eight years of regular use because of anxiety about possible side effects. The result was that the child spent seven weeks in hospital during the year, including a period when the eczema became infected.

A year later the eczema was as bad as ever and steroid treatment was resumed with the family's agreement. Before long the condition was much improved and the child's life much happier.

Although topical steroids vary considerably in strength, only the mildest steroid preparations are generally prescribed for babies and children, alternatives such as zinc or tar paste, or lubricating cream, being preferred (see below). The aim is to use them over very short periods of time, spreading small amounts thinly over the affected area. Even so, when the National Eczema Society was founded in 1975, it became obvious that the overwhelming cause for anxiety among patients and their families was the use of topical steroids.

At the time of writing, the Society is concerned about the DHSS decision to allow the mildest of these preparations (one per cent only of hydrocortisone) to be sold over the counter in five-gram tubes. Although a pharmacist must be present at the sale and can give advice, a doctor's prescription is no longer necessary. Doctors have asked manufacturers to enclose leaflets explaining the use and dangers of topical steroids. They are also monitoring any adverse effects from sales over the counter.

Hydrocortisone is the weakest of the steroid creams, varying from ½–2½ per cent, and this is the best type of preparation for long-term use, particularly in sensitive areas like the face and groin.

Hydrocortisone preparations are prescribed under many different names, including Efcortelan. There is a useful tar/hydrocortisone mixture called Tarcortin.

The practice of combining a steroid preparation with another constituent in an ointment is quite common. Where infection is present, steroid treatment can be combined with the use of an anti-infective agent and sometimes both are present in one ointment, for example Vioform-hydrocortisone. This type of preparation is available only on prescription.

These are some of the steroid preparations your doctor may prescribe for you:

- **mildly potent** Carbo-Cort, Dioderm, Gregoderm, Neo-Cortef, Timodine
- **moderately potent** Alphaderm, Eumovate, Haelan, Synandone, Trimovate, Ultradil
- **potent** Propaderm, Betnovate, Nerisone, Topilar, Metosyn, Ledercort, Diprosalic, Adcortyl
- **very potent** Propaderm Forte, Dermovate, Nerisone Forte, Synalar Forte, Halciderm.

Among products available without prescription, there are:

- **soothing creams/lotions** Alpha Keri, Diprobase, Eczederm (contains calamine), Natuderm, Sudocrem, Ultrabase
- **soothing creams** to which other substances can be added: emulsifying ointment (see under *Bathing* in this

chapter), white vaseline, Alcoderm, Unguentum Merck, E45 Boots (contains lanolin – see page 67), Clinitar
- **for the bath** Alpha Keri, Aveeno bath oil, Oilatum emollient and soaps – Aveeno bar, Simple
- **shampoos** Alphosyl application, Clinitar, Genisol.

Case history *John, now adult, illustrates features common to most instances where eczema is mild and quickly brought under control. At the same time, because it relates the facts about one individual, his case shows how much it is impossible to generalise about allergic illness.*

John was breast-fed until seven months but his mother does not know whether he was given a night-time formula based on cow's milk during their stay in a maternity unit.

Eczema developed at around five months. The earliest symptom appeared after a walk on the first mild day of spring. John was wearing woollen leggings and a mild rash was present when they were removed indoors. Untypically, it was on the front of both legs and there was no sign of reddening on any other part of his body. He began to scratch and what had been a mild condition became raw and bleeding. The family doctor seemed to regard the rash as trivial and the creamy liquid he prescribed proved impractical in use. Bandaging John's legs became a daily nightmare.

When solids were first introduced, the rash began to worsen. John did not seem to like eggs. A woollen cap left a red mark across his forehead and the rash spread to his hands and wrists. At this stage John's parents were referred to a local dermatologist who suggested a diet eliminating cow's milk and eggs, substituting a special milk formula then marketed for allergic children, and stressed that foods rich in iron and vitamins, liver, for example, must be given to take the place of eggs. The dermatologist expressed the opinion that John was unlikely to develop asthma.

From that point the eczema was well controlled with a mild hydrocortisone ointment and a tar preparation and by the age of two, John's eczema had disappeared. However, as a schoolboy he developed nasal congestion and as a teenager, asthma (see Chapter 5). Both conditions cleared up eventually, despite the fact that he became a heavy smoker as an adult.

John's asthma was always worse in the autumn and a visit to an allergist provided the explanation. Although not allergic to many pollens, he was highly sensitive to moulds present at that time of year. He also proved allergic to nuts (although not peanuts which belong to the pulse family), vomiting on more than one occasion, the last time so violently that he was careful to avoid them after that.

This case history – an instance where allergies were trouble-some, occasionally distressing but not generally severe – illustrates the type of anomalies which often occur in individual accounts. Eczema was worse on the front of the legs, hardly occurring at all on the face, which is often the first part of the body affected. The experienced dermatologist was wrong in predicting that it would not lead on to asthma in later life. Finally, the disappearance of John's asthma was unaffected by his increasingly heavy smoking, in direct contradiction to all accepted knowledge about the illness.

Many cases of childhood eczema are similar in pattern to John's, but some become more widespread and severe, presenting a different set of problems, both medical and emotional.

Case history *Alan, aged seven, suffered from severe eczema from the time he was a few months old. For medical reasons, his mother was unable to breast-feed for the first week of his life and believes that he must have been given a formula based on cow's milk in the maternity unit. There was no known history of allergy in the families of either parent.*

Once Alan was taken home at a week old, he was breast-fed for six months and his eczema started on weaning to a mixed diet. The rash was worst on his chest and back and the family GP referred him to a dermatologist at the local hospital. Alan was treated with a variety of steroid creams of varying potency. His mother was aware that this treatment could have harmful side effects and became anxious, particularly when some of the ointments seemed to make his skin condition worse.

The dermatologist conceded that diet might be partly responsible for his skin condition, but did not feel it would be useful to eliminate any foods. By this time, Alan was also suffering from asthma – and attending another specialist for this condition – as well as digestive problems including sickness and diarrhoea.

By the time he was two Alan was covered with eczema from head to foot. It was so severe on his neck that he could not turn his head for the pain. His mouth was so sore that he was eating very little. He bled freely yet continued scratching and it was evident that he was a very sick child. His mother then heard of the National Eczema Society and attended a meeting where a consultant discussed the importance of diet. Understanding her anxiety about Alan, her family doctor agreed to refer him to this specialist for a second opinion.

He was then admitted to hospital and a strict diet initiated in order to identify foods to which he was allergic. At the same time, the use of steroid creams was discontinued.

Alan proved to be allergic to many foods, including the soya milk which is tolerated by most atopic children. However, on a severely limited diet his skin began to clear up and as he grew older he was able to eat more and more different foods without ill effect. In place of cow's milk he now takes Pregestimil.

Although his eczema still flares up occasionally, it is well controlled and he lives a comparatively normal life, understanding that there are foods he must not eat. There have been two crises. On one occasion he had a mouthful of his brother's breakfast cereal and complained of the horrible taste of the milk. His mother realised immediately that he had taken the wrong plate. As a result he developed widespread urticaria (see Chapter 7) which subsided following a dose of antihistamine, prescribed by the doctor for such emergencies. On a second occasion, he played a toy mouth organ and said afterwards that his lips hurt. They began to swell grotesquely (angioedema – see Chapter 7) but once again the condition was controlled by the antihistamine. It is likely that the toy was made of nickel, known to be the most allergenic metal (see later in the chapter). However, it is clear that Alan's life will probably not be severely affected by his allergies because his family has a good understanding of them and emergencies can be dealt with promptly.

Case history This optimistic outlook for Alan can be contrasted with handicaps suffered by 37-year-old Michael who also suffered from severe eczema from babyhood. As he became older, it was accompanied by perennial rhinitis (see Chapter 6) and asthma (Chapter 5).

Out of a normal school life of ten years, he calculates that he *had no more than six years of regular attendance. Nobody ever suggested his sitting an examination. He spent long spells in a hospital ward occupied by skin and geriatric cases, both equally outcast. As he grew older, he failed to keep jobs because of constant illness.*

For the past year, he has adopted a wholefood diet for the first time with a marked improvement in his allergic illnesses. He has eliminated all dairy produce and beef. He drinks soya milk and eats wholemeal bread and can also tolerate some fruit and vegetables.

His skin still peels from the effect, he believes, of early steroid treatment. His second daughter was born with eczema covering her entire body, a rare occurrence. As her mother suffered from allergies as well, they knew that any children they had would be at high risk, but because they both now know a great deal about the condition, their daughter's skin is much improved and the outlook is hopeful.

Case histories of this kind emphasise the role played by food in atopic eczema, although there is still controversy on the subject among dermatologists. It may be that food is a much more important factor in some cases than others. Sometimes, a worsening of the skin condition has been observed within minutes of the food being eaten, but a response can take place up to a day or two later. Patients often appear to have a tolerance level so that, as an example, one glass of milk will not provoke a worsening of the symptoms, but several glasses over a period will do so. There is more about food allergy in Chapter 8.

Contact eczema (dermatitis)

In the context of this book, this is a 'rogue' disorder because it does not belong to the group including asthma, hay fever, urticaria and anaphylaxis – all Type I reactions – but to Type IV classification of delayed hypersensitivity (see Chapter 2). It has been included because it is a common skin disorder causing various degrees of discomfort and inconvenience.

The wide variety of substances concerned are known as 'contactants' and act as haptens (see Chapter 2) combining with protein in the skin to form a complete allergen. This means that the substance actually penetrates the skin, causing the symptoms of eczema.

Symptoms and diagnosis

The symptoms of contact dermatitis are similar to those of atopic eczema. The skin becomes red and very itchy with the formation of tiny blisters which weep as a result of scratching. Once the condition becomes chronic, the skin takes on a dry scaly appearance.

Although sensitisation can occur in seven to ten days after the first encounter with the contactant, more frequently the disorder develops after repeated and prolonged exposure. This is in very marked contrast to the form of contact allergy due to Type I reaction. The condition affects children more often than older patients. A rash develops around the mouth on contact with certain foods – those most likely to produce this somewhat rare effect are egg, tomato and orange.

Early diagnosis of true contact dermatitis – the word is in more common use than eczema (from Greek 'derma': skin; 'itis': inflammation) but they are interchangeable – is not difficult if the patient is seen shortly after the rash develops. Symptoms are present where the contact has taken place. In severe cases, the dermatitis may spread to cover wide areas of the body and can continue to increase in severity for up to seven days without further contact with the substance concerned.

In Chapter 2 it was explained that skin tests for allergies are not wholly consistent because results sometimes fail to correlate with the patients' symptoms. However, patch testing is reliable in identifying contactants involved in this type of dermatitis because it reproduces the conditions which caused the skin disorder in the first instance. For this reason, it is never undertaken during an acute phase of the disease because there is a risk of exacerbating the dermatitis.

Patch testing is usually carried out on the back to intact skin. Procedures, including the range of substances used, have been standardised internationally. Patients are given explicit instructions:

- leave the patches in place for 48 hours
- do not take a bath or shower or wash your back while the patches are in place
- avoid excessive exertion causing perspiration
- avoid rubbing the patches
- do not expose the back to sun
- if the patches come loose, re-stick them and inform the doctor that this has been done.

The suspected contactants are dissolved in petroleum jelly and the patches fixed to the back with a special adhesive tape which has been found unlikely to cause a reaction. If a plant is suspected as causing the rash, fresh leaves make an ideal testing material.

Allergens

Nickel, the most highly allergenic metal and used extensively in plating and alloys, is very often responsible for allergic reactions in women and girls, less frequently in men. Some people can react to it even through a layer of cloth. Approximately one in seven women over the age of eighteen is sensitive to nickel. Before 1968 the main cause of sensitivity was from suspenders and when these were replaced more and more by tights, dermatologists hoped that they might see a decrease in nickel allergy.

However, the increased popularity of ear piercing has given a boost to the incidence of this particular allergy. A 'gold-plated' nickel sleeper is enough to produce sensitivity and although the rash may be confined to the ear lobe, the entire skin becomes allergic to nickel.

The source of nickel allergy is quite easily identified from the site of the contact dermatitis:

- the scalp or side of the head – hairpins, curlers, spectacles

- the ears and surrounding area – clip-on earrings and inexpensive ones for pierced ears
- neck and chest – necklaces, lockets, medals, zips
- waistline – buckles and stud fastenings on jeans, skirts and shorts
- thighs – metal chairs, coins in pockets
- hands – taps, scissors, rings, thimbles, handles
- arms – watch straps, bracelets, arms of metal chairs
- feet – buckles, zips, shoe eyelets.

Case history *This is the case history of a young office worker who proved to be highly nickel-sensitive. Ironically, she was employed by the Royal Mint, but the only coins she handled in the course of her work were enclosed in capsules. Her first symptoms appeared when she was 20 after wearing a wrist watch. A red and extremely itchy rash appeared as a circle round her left wrist. She stopped wearing the watch and eventually the circle went away.*

A year or two later she developed a similar red and weeping rash on her right hand. Patch testing proved her highly sensitive to nickel: the test itself made her miserable because the nickel patch became very itchy. She was treated with steroid creams for a year but stopped using them because her skin began to thin.

The second reaction on her right hand occurred when she started handling money in the course of her work. Her specialist said that her only course was to avoid nickel in every form. This meant covering the handles of scissors; lacquering the handles of filing cabinets; avoiding paper clips and all inexpensive jewellery. Earrings have produced a local rash as well as making the rash on her hands flare up.

When the condition is really bad (it gets worse sometimes and she feels it is affected by stress) she wears cotton gloves. A number of other substances act as irritants including lanolin (see page 67), carbon paper and newsprint. The rash has damaged her nails and destroyed some of the cuticles.

Stainless steel contains five per cent nickel so a very large number of household fitments can affect sensitive individuals.

Both nurses and hairdressers are at special risk from nickel (scissors, surgical instruments); their jobs involve other substances which can cause contact dermatitis. For nurses, these include **local anaesthetics** and ethylenediamine, a preservative often added to ointments, including topical antihistamines. This means that one treatment in use for atopic and contact skin conditions can itself cause a harmful reaction. **Hair dyes** are a well-known source of skin disorders which is one reason why hairdressers wear gloves. Unfortunately, some of them may react to artificial rubber. Finally, both groups have their hands in water frequently, suffering the irritant effect of detergents and antiseptics.

Artificial rubber is a potent cause of contact dermatitis: gloves, sponges, shoes and even elastic can produce symptoms because of their rubber content. Once sensitised by a contactant, skin in any part of the body will produce a reaction to it. A woman with dermatitis on her forehead, caused by the elastic on her hairnet, one day chewed some bubblegum and suffered a severe reaction to her lips because she had not realised that artificial rubber could be a constituent of bubblegum.

Contact dermatitis is a common problem for people at work in many industrial environments. Special oils are used habitually in all processes involved in cutting metal and machine rooms often have a tub of **solvent** with which engineering workers clean their hands regularly. Prolonged use of this solvent can cause dermatitis, an effect which can be avoided if vaseline or a moisturising cream is applied before going to work and on returning home.

A phenomenon (reported by Dr Hindson of Sunderland's Royal Infirmary) is the young person whose principal symptom is a bright scarlet face. This is practically always the result of the modern habit of washing hair daily – common to both sexes – and is a reaction to formalin, a preservative found in most **shampoos**. The scalp itself is not involved because, in this instance, it seems to have an inherent lack of response (reported in *The Journal of the American Medical*

Association, 26.11.82). To these patients Dr Hindson recommends Head and Shoulders shampoo made by Procter and Gamble because it is free of formalin.

Chromate, the yellow colouring, can affect teachers, for instance, who use yellow chalk to write on blackboards, and workers in the tanning industry. Furniture lacquer, nail varnish and dyes used in many industries are other proven causes of contact dermatitis.

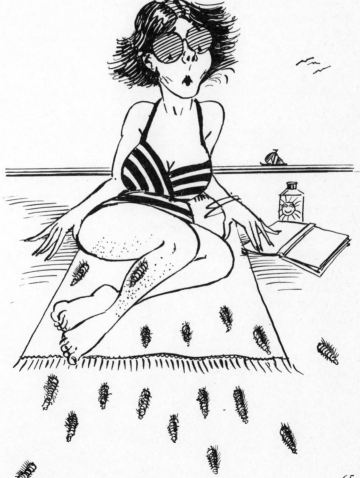

UA-3

Certain **plants** can cause symptoms in some people. The best known of these is the polyanthus, although tulip bulbs can also be troublesome. Poison ivy and poison oak, found in the USA but not in Europe, can cause very serious reactions.

A final example of the huge range of substances which have been found responsible for provoking contact dermatitis was reported in *The Sunday Times* in May 1984: a plague of black and red hairy caterpillars, larvae of the brown-tail moth, was reported to be sweeping across southeast England. The hairs were found to carry a chemical capable of causing rashes and even temporary blindness.

Treatment

Treatment for contact dermatitis is basically the same as for atopic eczema (see earlier in the chapter). The most important advice is, as always, avoid the allergen. For those at work, employment in another department may be possible; alternatively, gloves and protective clothing should be worn. After a serious outbreak, a patient should not return to work before the condition clears up: the skin acts as an essential barrier and once it is broken there is always the possibility of infection as a serious complication.

Topical steroids of the kind used for the treatment of atopic eczema are the most popular form of treatment. If the condition is severe and the hands and/or feet are involved, stronger steroid preparations may be necessary. Most commercial steroid preparations do not contain lanolin, a potential contactant, but some have neomycin, another known sensitiser: your doctor should prescribe something without these ingredients.

Irritant eczema

It is easy to confuse contact dermatitis with irritant eczema. Irritant eczema is very common in atopic individuals whereas contact dermatitis is more common in people who do not suffer from other allergies. Another difference is that contact dermatitis is often difficult to treat other than by avoidance of the allergen, whereas irritant eczema responds more readily to use of moisturising creams and the methods used for treating atopic eczema (see pages 56–57).

Wet cement is a common cause of irritant eczema. Damp conditions in such places as car washing systems or leather tanning can be poor environments for those at risk. Other substances capable of causing contact or irritant disorders include certain plastics, paints, glues, insulation and the waterproof finish applied to rainwear.

Cosmetics and perfumes are commonly the cause of this type of allergy. **Lanolin,** very often an ingredient of moisturising or soothing creams, can be implicated. It is not unusual for elderly people to use lanolin as a form of self-medication for varicose dermatitis (see overleaf) and in some cases there is no doubt that the lanolin exacerbates the condition, although some doctors feel that the extent to which this has been blamed has been exaggerated in the past. There are now a number of ranges of 'hypoallergenic' beauty products including Almay and the Clinique range. These are the best choice for anyone who has reacted to any of the numerous additives used in regular ranges. The Simple range of products is also made without perfume and is relatively inexpensive.

Other forms of dermatitis

There are many other forms of dermatitis in which allergy may or may not play a part. These are a few of the more common conditions.

Nummular eczema

The cause of this form is unknown and it is very difficult to treat. The red disc-shaped rash is mainly confined to the lower legs, sometimes to the lower arms. Occasionally, there is a history of childhood eczema, but very often the patient has never suffered from skin problems before. Tests for contact allergens are invariably negative.

Seborrhoeic dermatitis

The typical sufferer in this group is a man aged between 20 and 30. The disorder seems to be an adult version of an infant's 'cradle cap'. It occurs in parts of the body with a large number of grease-producing sebaceous glands including the scalp, face, chest and under the arms. The rash itself is insignificant but the patient finds it extremely uncomfortable and itchy. The cause is unknown and it is difficult to treat. Shaving is often a problem and the patient can find growing a beard the easiest course.

Varicose dermatitis

This is a disorder of the elderly and follows the development of varicose veins which result from a slowing up of the blood flow in the legs. A typical sufferer is an overweight, elderly woman who has had a number of pregnancies. The wearing of support tights or stockings combined with weight control can be sufficient to prevent the development of varicose veins.

However, once the condition is present the skin in the

area becomes thin and delicate. It may become inflamed and itchy and medical help should be asked for at this stage to prevent further complications. Once the skin breaks down as a result of scratching or continual knocks against a piece of furniture, there is a danger of developing a varicose ulcer. This is a very common disorder among elderly men and women and signals a long and wearisome period of pain and treatment before the ulcer heals.

It is important to follow treatment recommended by a doctor because contact dermatitis may develop as a result of using creams which have not been prescribed. Any ill effects from prescribed ointments – itching or inflammation for example – should be reported to the doctor at once.

Rashes as a result of drugs are not uncommon and these are dealt with in Chapter 10.

4
Eye and ear allergies

Where an allergic disorder is concerned, it is typical for one set of symptoms to predominate in one person, another set in another individual. For example, some may find tickling inside the nose, sneezing and watery discharge (hay fever) far more troublesome than anything else. Others suffer from asthma, particularly at night. For many, eye symptoms are the major concern.

A parent may not consider the possibility of allergy if a young child continually rubs at itchy eyes or complains of a 'blocked' sensation in one or both ears. Yet allergy can often be the cause of these uncomfortable symptoms and once it is correctly diagnosed, treatment usually proves effective.

Eyes

Each eyelid has an external layer of loosely bound skin, the thinnest in the body, with the result that swelling can occur very readily. The conjunctiva is a delicate mucous membrane lining the inside of both upper and lower eyelids, and extending over the front of the eye.

Allergists recognise that the external eye possesses a high degree of sensitivity and reacts to new allergens more readily than any other part of the body. For this reason, an eye challenge was sometimes used in the past instead of the more usual modern skin test when trying to isolate an allergen causing hay fever, for instance. A single sterile drop containing the suspected allergen was introduced into the eye and a positive reaction – reddening, watering and swelling – took place in the same interval generally observed for a skin test, ten minutes or less.

However, such is the sensitivity of the eyes that a very severe reaction occurred in some cases, so eye challenge fell into disuse. As well as causing considerably less discomfort, skin testing has the advantage that many allergens can be employed in one session, while only one substance at a time can be tested with an eye challenge.

In general, allergic reactions affecting the eye are less common in children than in adults. However, eye problems are not unusual in cases of infantile eczema.

Allergic conjunctivitis

This condition (the inflammation of the conjunctiva) is the most common reaction. Symptoms include extreme itchiness, reddening, watering, and sometimes swelling which may be slight but can be so severe that the eye is distorted in an alarming way. Occasionally, the condition occurs in babies: a milky white swelling protrudes between the eyelids. This is particularly distressing for parents as the symptom appears suddenly and the allergen responsible is very difficult to trace. Fortunately, the condition responds well to treatment with antihistamine.

Severe itching with inevitable rubbing of the eyes almost always indicates that conjunctivitis is allergic in origin. The sufferer may experience some pain and photophobia (sensitivity to light) on waking. Watery discharge is general, but if the eyelids are stuck together after sleep and there is thick mucus and crusted material on the lashes, infection is present.

Allergic conjunctivitis is often seen in older children with hay fever and the same air-borne allergens, pollens, dusts and moulds, for example, can be responsible for both conditions. As these are blown into the eyes, it is a sensible precaution for those at risk to wear protective sunglasses out of doors.

However, following original sensitisation by such allergens, similar symptoms can appear as a result of other antigens, food being one example. Occasionally, allergic conjunctivitis may be the only symptom of food allergy.

Vernal conjunctivitis

This is a more serious recurrent disease affecting most patients between the ages of six and twenty (from Latin 'vernalis': spring) but it is nevertheless very rare. Three times as many boys as girls suffer from it. These patients show similar positive results to the standard investigations for allergy (see Chapter 2) – skin testing, RAST and evidence of histamine (this has even been found in the tears of some sufferers).

There is a great deal of evidence that vernal conjunctivitis is an atopic disorder. In one group of 35 patients seen in an allergy clinic:

- 68 per cent had eczema
- 63 per cent had hay fever
- 63 per cent had asthma
- only 14 per cent had no associated allergic disease.

Summer was the worst season for more than half the patients, spring for more than one-third while the rest reported no detectable seasonal influence. Of the total number, 79 per cent were male and 76 per cent less than ten years old at the time of referral. The most common allergens were animal danders and grass pollens.

The symptoms of vernal conjunctivitis can be shortlived but they can also last for months or become inactive for a few months before reappearing. In addition to redness of the eye and severe itching, sufferers experience severe photophobia (see above) and a heavy, thick discharge.

Another feature of the disease is the appearance of a 'cobblestone' effect of wart-like protuberances inside the upper eyelid. These can be quite small or massive and in some cases there may be formation of ulcers on the cornea (the transparent 'window' at the front of the eye through which light passes); these heal but can leave scarring. The 'cobblestone' effect is not in itself harmful. However, if the disease reactivates, there is increased swelling, inflammation and discomfort. The risk of serious eye infection is greater when the onset of the disorder is late – in teenagers and adults.

In recent years, a similar condition exhibiting the 'cobblestone' effect has been reported in an increasing number of patients (some children among them) who wear contact lenses. Among symptoms experienced are mild itching, the production of mucus and eventually an inability to continue wearing the lenses. There is never damage to the cornea, but some patients find the symptoms so intolerable that they have to stop wearing lenses altogether. Sometimes the lens itself has been implicated (more commonly the soft type than the hard) and on other occasions the preparations used for cleaning and sterilising – changing to new fluid should then ease the symptoms.

Treatments

Allergy-induced conjunctivitis ranges from a mild ailment to a much more serious condition which can even threaten the sight. Simple allergic conjunctivitis responds well to antihistamine eyedrops, for example Vasocon-A and Otrivine-Antistin. These reduce itching and swelling. If they prove inadequate a sodium cromoglycate preparation, Opticrom, may be more effective.

When the condition is more serious, however, the mainstay of therapy is topical steroids. As this condition waxes and wanes, treatment should be confined to periods when the disease is active, as the use of steroids – particularly where young children are concerned – is always potentially dangerous.

In allergic eye conditions, it is important to wash the hands frequently to prevent infecting the eyes by rubbing.

Ears

Secretory otitis media (SOM)

This is the most common ear disorder of childhood. SOM is simply an inflammation of the middle ear with the formation of fluid. The part played by allergy is the subject of controversy, but there is increasing evidence that food allergy in particular may well be a contributing factor. An ear examination is a sensible precaution to take if a child suffers from hay fever or asthma. Ear ache is not necessarily a symptom (although some hearing loss often is) and the condition can be overlooked easily.

In a typical Ear, Nose and Throat (ENT) unit, SOM is responsible for around sixty per cent of the surgery on children under ten. The condition causes an unnatural accumulation of fluid behind the ear drum; this forms if the air is unable to pass easily from the nose through the Eustachian tube into the middle ear. The tube normally opens when swallowing, yawning or chewing takes place, but becomes blocked and unable to open if the adenoids are enlarged or tissues in the area are swollen. As swelling is one of the principal features of allergy, it is possible that allergy causes – or at least exacerbates – the condition.

A surgeon removes fluid from the middle ear by placing a small tube through the ear drum. This may be extremely difficult because the fluid can be thick and viscous. In some cases the operation is repeated a number of times because fluid re-forms once the tube is removed.

The symptoms of SOM are:

- hearing loss, mild or severe, which may be continuous or intermittent
- pain or discharge from the ear
- a feeling of blockage
- ringing or crackling sounds.

Symptoms normally start between the ages of two and six and boys are twice as likely to be affected as girls.

One study quoted in *Allergy – immunological and clinical aspects*, edited by Professor M H Lessof, showed a link between breast-feeding and SOM. The mothers of 256 babies were encouraged to breast-feed for as long as possible; examinations of the children were carried out until the age of three. In the first year, 19 per cent of the babies who were breast-fed for less than two months developed otitis and after three years the figure rose to 26 per cent. Of those who were breast-fed for more than six months, only six per cent developed SOM in the first year and the figure remained at that level two years later. Bottle-fed babies are more likely to regurgitate milk to the middle ear via the nasal passages, which could provoke otitis.

Another investigation (quoted in the same book) showed that 48 per cent of children who developed SOM came from families with a history of the condition. Improvement took place when specific allergens were eliminated from the diet, with a relapse when they were reintroduced. The most common allergens proved to be cow's milk, eggs, chicken, chocolate, corn, wheat and – among inhalants – house dust, pollens, moulds, feathers and cat dander.

It has been observed that the site of allergic reaction can vary according to the season. For example a child under seven who has hay fever during the summer months may also suffer from SOM then.

Referral to an ENT unit is essential if there is any suspicion that a child's hearing is abnormal. Slight hearing loss is often difficult to detect but if a child cannot hear the ticking of a watch held close to either ear, the parent should seek professional advice.

There are, however, many reasons for poor hearing. Infection and excessive ear wax are examples and hearing often improves after tonsils and adenoids are removed. However, when hay fever or asthma are present it is possible that ear symptoms are allergic in origin. Very often infection is also present and medication to deal with this aspect is then prescribed.

5
Asthma

In past centuries, asthma was considered a disease of the intelligent, sensitive and well-born. The reason may well have been that this group was able to obtain the best medical attention, while a touch of wheezing was accepted by the poor as a small part of their heavy burden, and therefore disregarded.

Like all allergic conditions, asthma is capricious. It can vary in severity and then disappear for years, only to re-appear – all without discernible reason. Yet the days when the asthmatic child was regarded as frail and 'weak-chested', unable to take part in any vigorous activity, are long gone.

Many distinguished people in various walks of life have been asthmatics for a part – at least – of their lives. The former Labour Party leader Michael Foot MP revealed that his attacks began at university, triggered by clouds of builders' dust. The attacks waned some years later when all his ribs were broken in a car accident. Asthmatics have become Olympic gold medallists and Christopher Reeve, the screen 'Superman', is known to suffer from asthma.

Statistics

Asthma can be divided into three categories:

- 'extrinsic' or atopic – caused by allergies – which is the type affecting most children and 50 per cent of adults
- 'intrinsic' – due to other causes such as infection – which affects more adults; it is less well understood

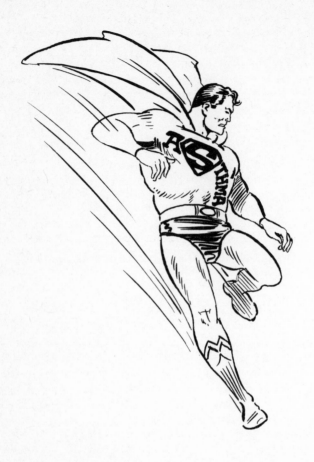

- attacks induced by sensitivity to drugs, notably aspirin (see Chapter 10).

'Intrinsic' asthma typically develops in later life and frequently becomes chronic. It may be an atopic disorder in some cases. It is often exacerbated by infection in the sinuses. Features of both atopic and intrinsic asthma may be present in the same person.

Asthma is the major allergic disease of childhood. It has

been estimated that about one in ten children and one in twenty adults in the UK suffers from allergic asthma. (While allergy is the cause of most asthma in childhood, it is responsible for only about 50 per cent of the disease in adults.) Of the two million asthmatics in the UK, fifty per cent experience their first symptoms before they are five. It is twice as common in boys up to 14 and it is they who have the more serious symptoms.

Yet, despite the vast array of modern drugs available to control everything from a comparatively mild condition to a crisis which can threaten life, asthma remains a serious and distressing illness. It is responsible for more absence from school than any other chronic disease. In the USA, for instance, of all the school days lost each year to illness or injury, about 60 per cent are because of asthma and other acute respiratory conditions.

Among many widely held misconceptions about asthma is that it is never fatal. The Asthma Research Council reported 1,954 deaths in the UK from the illness in 1984 (all ages). On the other hand, it is reassuring to know that most children grow out of asthma, although not invariably. In a recent study of 267 children, followed up for more than 20 years, it was shown that:

- 52 per cent became almost completely free of symptoms
- 21 per cent had one or two episodes a year
- 27 per cent had remissions for at least three years
- 7 children died, three during attacks of asthma.

Professor Margaret Turner-Warwick of the Cardiothoracic Institute and London's Brompton Hospital believes that two-thirds of deaths from asthma can be attributed to poor understanding on the part of doctors and patients. Reported in *Asthma News* (published by the Asthma Society and Friends of the Asthma Research Council), she said: 'Deaths are fortunately very rare but the number is not yet falling and this seems to be because people are not sufficiently aware of the danger.' She added that many doctors were slow to understand their patients because they saw them only when they were relatively well and did not believe that they could get sudden and severe asthma attacks. Often patients knew more about their asthma than their doctors.

It is an interesting feature of the disease that the incidence varies a great deal from country to country. In 1961, tests carried out on 286 islanders from Tristan da Cunha showed that at least 32 per cent had asthma. Because Tristan is so isolated the population is highly inbred. In contrast, asthma is unknown in children and rare in adults in the Papua New Guinea highlands where the community would seem to be just as isolated as that on Tristan. Asian children also seem to have low incidence of the disease, whether born overseas or in the UK (but see page 33).

What happens during an asthma attack?

During an attack of asthma the lungs cease to function in the fashion most people take for granted. The main job of the lungs is to transfer oxygen from the air to the blood. Oxygen is then carried by the bloodstream to every part of the body, where it combines with glucose which is broken down chemically to release energy. The result of this energy reaction is the production of another gas, carbon dioxide, which is carried in the blood back to the lungs and then exhaled. For an easy interchange of oxygen and carbon dioxide to take place, the lungs must function freely without obstruction. This does not happen during an asthmatic attack.

The mechanism of atopic asthma can be explained as a classic response of Type I allergic reaction (see Chapter 2). The foreign substance, the allergen, is recognised by the immune system and as a result, IgE antibodies specific to it are produced. Very little IgE is released into the blood: most of it clings to mast cells in the airways and lungs. When the allergen is inhaled again it meets mast cells coated with specific IgE antibody. Antibody and allergen combine, resulting in breakdown of the mast cell which releases a variety of chemicals which cause the allergic reaction.

Eosinophils, a type of white blood cell that regulates inflammation, fill the airways. The lungs become over-inflated, with air being left behind even after exhaling. Asthmatics commonly find breathing out more difficult than breathing in. As a result, there is a build-up of carbon dioxide and an urgent desire for fresh air.

Symptoms can vary considerably, and there is a small group whose only symptom is a cough, but even if the attack is comparatively mild, the first symptom is often a feeling of discomfort in the chest. Many patients follow up with a dry cough, soon accompanied by wheezing and breathlessness due to obstructed airways as the smooth muscles surrounding them contract.

Wheezing, only detectable when the sufferer breathes out forcibly in the early stages, can later also be heard when he breathes in. He becomes restless, agitated and fearful, and coughing increases. At first the cough may be unproductive but as it worsens, many asthmatics start being able to cough up sputum. Sometimes, especially if infection is present as an additional complication, this can literally plug the bronchial passages.

At the height of an attack, the skin is clammy and the sufferer looks pale and anxious. Sitting leaning forward with the elbows on the knees is a typical posture. Asthmatics never want to lie down because in that position breathing seems more difficult. Speech is very often impossible and a severe attack can be so exhausting that the patient is unable to walk even a short distance. The skin may appear blue because of lack of oxygen in the blood. Wheezing eventually abates but unfortunately this final symptom can be misinterpreted to mean that the patient's condition is improving. In fact, it is a sign that obstruction of the airways has worsened to such an extent that breathing becomes soundless. The converse is true – as a patient improves wheezing will be resumed.

Not all asthmatic episodes are as severe as this. Indeed, it is possible to wheeze without having asthma, but equally not all asthmatics wheeze. Many people do so occasionally with infection and have no need to fear that it heralds the onset of asthma.

Moreover, several patterns of asthma are known to exist. Immediate Type I reaction as described above begins within minutes of exposure to the inhalant, peaks within 30 minutes and subsides after an hour. In late asthma, airway obstruction does not begin until one hour or later after exposure, becomes progressively worse at a gradual rate and is often more severe than the immediate variety.

The symptoms, whether mild or severe, occur in paroxysms. The airways are extremely sensitive to irritants which may not always be allergens known to affect the individual. Wheezing can occur as a result of coughing, laughter, a change of environment or the fumes of such thing as petrol, wood smoke or cigarette smoke.

Causes

Asthma can begin in infancy, frequently starting when a baby has a lung infection or flu or after measles. Very often it is the babies who succumb to eczema, colic or allergy-induced 'constant colds' who show the earliest signs of asthma.

In Nottingham, Dr R Henry has had a special interest for many years in the pre-school child, of whom between 15 and 20 per cent wheeze. Some of his findings were published in *Asthma News* in 1985. One result confirmed that acute **bronchiolitis**, an infection of the bronchioles (tiny airways which form a network inside the lungs), can often lead on to the development of asthma which may persist.

Bronchiolitis is the most serious chest infection in the first year of life, affecting between one to two per cent of babies. The Nottingham team followed up children for four years after they had recovered and discovered that 75 per cent went on to develop further attacks of coughing and wheezing. The team is now trying to find out whether the children were born with a tendency to asthma, with bronchiolitis just the first manifestation. If this hypothesis proves accurate, it may be possible to prevent asthma in a significant number of children. Vaccines are now under development which may protect babies against bronchiolitis.

A few wheezes do not constitute asthma. Recurrent attacks, very often accompanied by other atopic disorders, are essential before a firm diagnosis of asthma can be made. In adults, **bronchitis** presents a similar range of symptoms and infection can trigger asthma in adults just as it does in children.

Pets Occasionally, it is easy to identify the allergen causing asthmatic symptoms. For example, a family acquires a cat as a pet for the first time. Shortly afterwards a child in the household develops a slight cough and a feeling of tightness in the chest. After the child fondles the animal, the mild symptoms are followed by wheezing and distress.

Cats are the animal most likely to produce a Type I allergic reaction when their hair and dander (tiny particles of skin) are inhaled. The dander remains in a room, even one that has been thoroughly cleaned, for long after the pet has left. All members of the cat family – leopards, tigers, lions and jaguars – have been known to affect zoo attendants, circus performers and vets in this way. The saliva of animals can also cause an allergic reaction in the form of urticaria where they have licked the skin – see Chapter 7.

Pet gerbils were identified as the cause of asthma and hay fever in three instances reported in *Clinical Allergy* in 1985. Allergy was confirmed by skin tests and RAST (see Chapter 2) and the cure effected when contact with the animals ceased. A Leeds survey in 1976 suggested that rodents were the most popular household pet and gerbils accounted for 61 per cent of the total. Gerbils, as well as hamsters, rats, mice and guinea pigs, are used extensively in research laboratories, and sometimes give rise to severe symptoms in workers who handle them. Many other animals can be responsible for allergic reaction including horses, dogs, rabbits, sheep, cows and budgerigars.

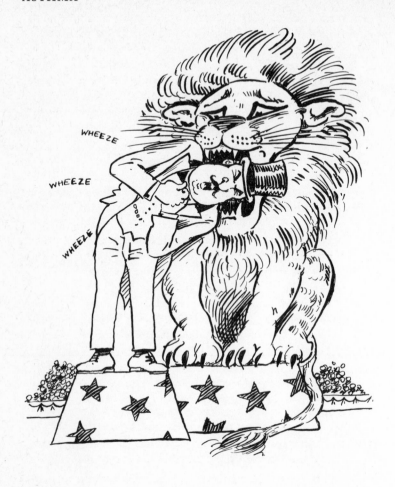

Unfortunately, it is seldom that the cause of asthma can be pinpointed with accuracy. Inhaled allergens, generally thought of in connection with hay fever, can be equally implicated in asthma, by far the more serious condition. They are very numerous and include a wide variety of pollens (most importantly those of trees and grasses), mites contained in house dust and moulds of many kinds.

The seasonal character of attacks can give a clue to the type of allergen involved. **Trees** pollinate in the UK between February and June so may be responsible for attacks at what would generally be regarded as a most untypical time of year. Hazel, for example, pollinates from January to April.

Spring grass begins to pollinate in April and is one of the earliest to shed its tiny grains into the gusty spring air. It is the many ripening **grasses** during May, June and July which make this period the height of the hay fever season (see Chapter 6). Dr A W Frankland, a leading allergist formerly at St Mary's Hospital, Paddington, has referred to 'Wimbledon fortnight reaction'. **Cereal pollens** must not be forgotten, usually affecting farm workers from June to September.

Flowers are not generally the source of much trouble although a few, including chrysanthemums, golden rod and wallflowers, may be responsible for asthma/hay fever symptoms.

Moulds and fungi are also important to the allergist although they are less known to the general public. They can often cause symptoms when there is no pollen in the air. Some occur on vegetables and others on cereal crops. One curious member of this group is *Serpula lacrimans*, causing dread in home owners although not many realise that it can also be responsible for their asthma – it is commonly known as **dry rot**.

House dust could well be the major cause of allergic asthma. Originally it was thought responsible for both asthma which had no seasonal pattern and perennial rhinitis (hay fever that persists all year). Now it is known that the real culprit is the house-dust mite (or perhaps its droppings), *Dermatophagoides pteronyssinus*, which lives on moulds and the tiny particles of skin shed by human bodies. Most beds have around 10,000 of these creatures. They are also liberally distributed in all living areas and an investigation reported in *Clinical Allergy* in 1985 showed that significant numbers are present in the beds of family pets.

All these substances are known allergens, but it is very seldom that one or a number of them is wholly responsible for an attack of asthma. Atopic people are known to have a high amount of IgE present in the skin which may be the reason that so many give positive reactions to a large number of potential allergens. It does not necessarily follow that they will react to the particular substance when they inhale it.

As well as reacting to allergens, asthmatics are very sensitive to **irritant inhalants** such as tobacco smoke, air pollution and fumes from gas boilers. Paint and paint thinner, perfumes, hairsprays and newsprint can also cause problems. The presence of static electricity has even been incriminated because it may attract allergens – pollens or spores for example – on to carpets and upholstery.

As well as all these common inhaled allergens the adult asthmatic encounters many potentially harmful substances at work. In the USA it has been estimated that up to 15 per cent of adult men developing asthma do so as a result of their work environment. It is recognised that workers with a history of atopy develop symptoms after a short period and with greater severity than non-atopic individuals.

In the UK a number of chemicals are recognised agents for occupational asthma as a prescribed industrial disease. These include:

- isocyanates – used for making plastic foam, synthetic inks, paints and adhesives
- platinum salts – used in platinum refining and found in laboratories
- acid anhydride and amine hardening agents – used for making adhesives, plastics, moulding resins and surface coatings
- soldering flux fumes from resin – used in the electronics industry
- enzymes in biological washing powders, baking, brewing – used in the food, fish and leather industries

- animals or insects – used for education or research purposes
- grain meal or flour dust (barley, oats, rye, wheat or maize) found on farms – used in the baking and milling industries.

Drugs (notably aspirin) can trigger attacks of asthma – this aspect is dealt with in Chapter 10 on drug allergies. Food allergy may well cause asthma alone, and it can exacerbate an attack. Food colourings, notably tartrazine (see Chapter 8), have been reported to cause asthma in aspirin-sensitive patients. Many other factors can play a role in provoking asthma. The most important are exercise, wind and temperature variations, emotion and infection (see later in the chapter). In adults, overwork, stress resulting from enforced unemployment, difficult relationships, and the responsibility of caring for children or the aged are all known triggers.

Diagnosis

The first essential – as with all allergies – is to compile a **detailed case history**. Some clinics produce their own charts. Others are available from companies which manufacture allergy solutions used in skin tests. Charts make sure that a very wide range of relevant information – including details about home environment, hobbies, animal contacts and family history as well as facts about the onset of symptoms – is laid out in an orderly fashion. It may be necessary to fill in charts over a period of months before a discernible pattern to the illness can be seen. Sometimes even then the capricious nature of allergic illness and the many provoking factors will make it impossible to recognise an overall design. However, well-compiled charts give valuable clues about which skin tests are most likely to prove positive.

Skin testing (see Chapter 2) is the method used most often in the diagnosis of inhalant allergies. For example, if your asthma attacks are worst during April and May it is very likely that you will prove to be allergic to tree pollens.

Some doctors are unconvinced of the value of skin testing. Atopic individuals often have a high level of IgE antibodies present in the skin and give positive weal and flare reactions to many substances. They may not suffer allergic symptoms to all the same substances. However, skin tests are generally regarded as a valuable part of the diagnosis of allergies.

The doctor will examine you carefully – ears, eyes and nose as well as throat. In order to assess the degree of bronchial obstruction due to narrowing of the airways, you will be asked to blow into a **spirometer** to measure what is known as 'vital capacity' (VC) – the volume of air which can be expelled from lungs after a deep breath; this device also charts the time taken to expel the breath. If lung function is normal, 70 per cent or more of total VC will be blown out in one second. An asthmatic will deliver 50 per cent or even as little as 20 per cent of the expelled breath in that time.

Another simple and useful device is the **peak flow meter** which also measures the rate at which air can be forced out of the lungs. Domestic versions of the meter which can be used effectively by young children are available. The meter measures 'peak expiratory flow rate' (PEFR) and enables a patient to keep a constant check on breathing performance. Very often symptoms are worst at night when the doctor is not on hand to witness them. If a record of peak flow can be kept on a 24-hour basis it can provide the doctor with a much more accurate picture of the waxing and waning of the condition. The fluctuations in the narrowing of the airways from hour to hour is a symptom typical to asthma and does not occur in bronchitis. Very often, reduced peak flow can give warning of an attack even before you begin to feel breathless. 'Morning dipping' of peak flow is common: it may well occur because lying in bed seems to make constriction of the airways worse for an asthmatic, who invariably prefers to sit up during the most severe attacks.

Bronchial challenge is a procedure which exposes a patient to a potentially allergenic material and then monitors the consequences. Because late reactions can result, it is standard practice to observe a patient for at least 48 hours after challenge. An increasing use is being made of bronchial challenge in order to assess the sensitivity of a patient's airways. Responses to given doses of histamine or methacholine can be measured. The latter is a substance which can provoke bronchial symptoms in a healthy person if it is given in a very high concentration. More on this can be found in Chapter 2.

Treatment

Once a diagnosis of asthma has been confirmed and the allergens identified, the first step must be to arrange the asthmatic's life so that as many trigger substances as possible can be avoided.

Suggestions to reduce the mite population – given that the sufferer is severely asthmatic and has a positive skin reaction to dust – are likely to delight only the most obsessive cleaners and polishers. They include:

- bedding, preferably made of synthetic materials because the mite has a preference for wool and cotton, should be washed weekly
- feathers, down or flock in pillows or duvet should be avoided
- a vacuum cleaner should be used daily on upholstery, curtains, mattress and blankets, and always under the bed, as well as on carpets
- curtains should be washed at least once every six weeks
- a damp duster should be used daily
- whenever possible, bedding should be put out of doors and sheets and pillowcases dried in the sun.

Although there is no scientific proof that dust extractors are useful, it can be reassuring to have one in the bedroom, particularly if pollens and moulds are among the allergens concerned. Humidifiers may do more harm than good because dust mites thrive in a warm, damp atmosphere; this also encourages the development of moulds and bacteria which can cause allergic reactions. (At the other extreme, the hot, dry atmosphere of a sauna is unlikely to be helpful either.) There is no scientific evidence that ionisers help asthmatics although this form of treatment has been used in the USSR for a number of years.

No one in the household should smoke and visitors should be discouraged from doing so. It is best to have no pets at all. Many foods cause wheezing within a few minutes so it is not difficult to identify those concerned. However, some foods can also produce a delayed reaction so are less easily traced (see Chapter 8).

It is impossible to eradicate all provoking agents – allergens, air pollutants, climate changes, emotional factors and infection – and symptoms are likely to persist without medication.

Caring for a severely asthmatic child at home calls for particular patience and good sense. Even if attacks are not provoked by excitement or distress, they will inevitably worsen if the child senses a high degree of anxiety in adults. There are a number of commonsense measures to follow in a severe attack of asthma:

- keep the child in his or her bedroom, which is always as clean as possible
- although no one with an attack of asthma will be able to eat or sleep, give plenty of fluid – a full glass every hour if possible. This can be a warm drink or soup – either of which will feel reassuring and may help to thin down the mucus and make it easier to cough up
- start medication at the earliest sign of wheezing: watch for individual symptoms of the onset of an attack – a slight cough, for example
- if treatment does not help within 30 minutes and breathing becomes so difficult that the patient is gasping, send for the doctor or take the child to an Accident and Emergency (casualty) department.

Parents must keep outwardly calm and can achieve this best if they understand what is happening to the child and know exactly what to do in a variety of circumstances. An extensive variety of medication, some free of side effects, others potentially dangerous, is now available. Prescribed and used sensibly, they can control even a severe attack – although there may be occasions when it is essential to get medical help.

Physiotherapists may help a patient by teaching him a technique known as 'postural drainage' which assists effective coughing up. Breathing exercises can also be helpful, not to strengthen chest muscles, which are often stronger than average in the asthmatic, but to learn a slow, deep method with the emphasis on breathing out. Breathing out is more difficult than breathing in during an attack and the build-up of air can lead to distension of the lungs with accompanying discomfort.

Medication

Sodium cromoglycate (SCG – Intal)
SCG was first isolated by the Fisons team in 1965. Dr Roger Altounyan was investigating the properties of a Middle Eastern plant from which the ancient Egyptian remedy 'khellin' was derived. Khellin was used to relieve breathing difficulties and seemed to have the ability to open up congested airways.

Dr Altounyan showed that it had powerful anti-allergenic properties. Intal is a prophylactic drug (from Greek 'pro': before; 'phulasso': guard) which means that it has to be taken regularly in order to prevent attacks of asthma. It has proved particularly effective in the treatment of children and in breathing difficulties as a result of exercise (see later in the chapter). Its side effects seem to be negligible.

SCG has no direct ability to open up narrowed airways and no antihistamine or anti-inflammatory properties. Studies have shown that the drug works by preventing the release of chemicals from mast cells: it forms a 'skin' around these cells, dispersing within a short period. This would explain why Intal has to be taken regularly in order to prevent attacks of asthma. It is not effective once an attack is in progress.

Used regularly, Intal has often been found to prevent recurrent attacks. It is available in aerosol form, and many asthmatics find this method the most convenient. It can also be taken as a dry powder inhaled through the mouth from a Spinhaler. This device must be used correctly: when asthmatics find Intal of little use, the reason may be that they are not taking it regularly enough or in the right way. Another reason may be that the initial dose has been insufficient. When good control has been established, many doctors reduce the dosage and cut down the frequency of use to three times daily, then to twice, as long as there is no reappearance of asthma. Some people, children in particular, find that Intal gives them a dry sore throat, so it is a good idea for them to drink something after using the Spinhaler.

(SCG has been used in a number of studies involving other allergies, those of the nose and eye, for example. There is increasing evidence that it is useful in a number of conditions.)

Steroids

When regular Intal, used four or six times daily, has not managed to control attacks, steroids (more properly known as corticosteroids) have to be considered. As in the case of severe atopic eczema (see Chapter 3), steroids are powerful, even life-saving, drugs. Recent research suggests that they protect against late as well as immediate reactions. They also increase the effectiveness of bronchodilators (see opposite). They can be inhaled from an aerosol, swallowed as tablets, or injected. Parents are understandably anxious if steroid treatment is prescribed for a child. However, the possible hazards are now well appreciated and the development of steroid aerosols means that the drug can be taken in very small amounts while remaining supremely effective and lessening the risk of side effects (see also Chapter 2).

Adults are at less risk from the side effects of steroids, even when taken by mouth, than children. The exact mechanism by which steroids work in the treatment of severe allergies is not understood although they have been in use for more than 30 years now. Their potency varies considerably. Whether the steroids are given by mouth or by injection, the response to a single dose starts after about two hours and peaks at around eight hours. Complete restoration of normal lung function can take anything from a few days to a week or longer.

Steroids in relatively high doses can also be most effective in controlling severe chronic asthma. Sometimes patients have been mis-diagnosed – as having chronic bronchitis, for example (where obstructed airflow is irreversible) – until steroid treatment is begun. It is then revealed that the airflow obstruction can be reversed, confirming a diagnosis of asthma.

Wherever possible, steroids taken in aerosol form are to be preferred to tablets (see above). There are patients, however, who can be maintained on oral steroids taken as a single dose every other day.

Where symptoms are less severe, many people find the use of bronchodilators sufficient to treat them.

Bronchodilators

These drugs have the effect of dilating or 'opening up' the narrowed airways which feature in an attack of asthma. Ephedrine, known to the ancient Chinese, belongs to this group, as does adrenaline, a potent drug that may save the life of a patient with a very severe attack of asthma – or reverse the symptoms of the most serious allergic reaction of all, anaphylactic shock (see Chapter 9). Adrenaline is the chemical produced in the adrenal glands upon vigorous exercise. It opens up the airways to make panting easier and switches blood circulation to the muscles so that the body is prepared for action. Many alternative bronchodilators have been developed which do not produce the powerful side effects associated with ephedrine and adrenaline – they open up the airways without the same powerful effects on other parts of the body.

The most commonly prescribed bronchodilators are fenoterol (Berotec), salbutamol (Ventolin) and terbutaline (Bricanyl). They may come in tablet, syrup, inhaler, aerosol and nebuliser forms but are most popular as an inhaler or aerosol. The drug is prepared so that under pressure in its canister it is liquid but when released it vaporises into tiny droplets which can be inhaled by mouth straight into the lungs.

This method of administering drugs produces more rapid relief than anything which has to be swallowed. Because it reaches the airways so rapidly, smaller doses are required than when taking oral medication and there is reduced likelihood of side effects. Normally one or two puffs from an aerosol are taken at any one time, each puff taken on a separate breath.

A child has to be taught carefully to use an inhaler because breathing in and pressing the canister must be coordinated. Sometimes a tube can be fitted to the aerosol (available for Bricanyl) to make the process easier.

The effect of an inhaler should last several hours. Asthmatic children are advised to use them when their chests feel tight and some may have to do so only occasionally. Others may need to use them regularly during the day to keep free of symptoms. A dose taken before some special event, particularly if it involves physical effort, will allow some children to take part in team games without developing symptoms.

An inhaler contains approximately 200 puffs so at a double dose of two puffs daily one should last for at least six weeks. If the aerosol is needed often to prevent an attack of asthma, a child should carry one with him. It is important for parents to explain to the staff at school how necessary the use of an aerosol may be to a child.

Some doctors do not like aerosols because they feel that both children and adults tend to over-use them. There was a rise in the rate of death from asthma in the 1960s which was believed to be associated with a particular drug (isoprenaline) no longer used in the UK.

The drugs used in nebulisers are the same as those employed in aerosols but they are dissolved in a salt solution enabling a much larger dose to be administered than would be possible from an aerosol. In the UK nebulisers are used in hospitals and occasionally supplied on loan to people whose asthma cannot be controlled in any other way.

Asthma News has printed the following warning about the use of nebulisers:

- no patient should buy one for his or her own treatment without reference to an asthma specialist
- if a nebuliser is not effective within 15 minutes a doctor should be called or the patient taken to the Accident and Emergency (casualty) department of a hospital
- assessment with various doses should be carried out before regular nebuliser treatment begins.

Although bronchodilators are best given by inhalation, there is one group of drugs for relaxing the bronchial tubes which has not yet been prepared in aerosol form. The best known of these drugs are:

- aminophylline (Phyllocontin, Theodrox)
- theophylline (Labophylline, Lasma, Nuelin, Pro-Vent, Slo-Phyllin, Theo-Dur, Theograd, Theosol, Uniphyllin).

These can be taken as tablets, capsules or a syrup. Unfortunately they can cause stomach irritation so are sometimes given as suppositories − a quick-acting method of administering drugs which is more popular in Europe than the UK.

In some severe attacks of asthma, none of these preparations may give speedy and lasting relief. Several bronchodilators, including aminophylline, salbutamol and terbutaline, can be injected by a doctor directly into the bloodstream or (sometimes) into muscle. Given this way, the drugs act very effectively.

Other factors

Infection

It is well known that viral infections (very often the common cold) play a major part in triggering asthma attacks. In children the earliest bout of wheezing often occurs when there is infection present.

Bronchitis produces symptoms very similar to those of asthma although it is caused by infection not allergy.

Asthmatic bronchitis usually means that a patient has episodes of asthma associated with bronchitis.

Exercise

It was known in the seventeenth century that exercise could provoke an attack in susceptible individuals, and there has until recently been a general belief that all exercise is bad for young asthmatics.

In the last decade, however, a scientific study has been made of exercise-induced asthma (EIA): it is now known to occur in 85 per cent of the children suffering from severe asthma. The 'short, sharp shock' regime, counselled by the Government in 1984 for young offenders, has been criticised as 'inhumane' for severe asthmatics since exercise in the cold is quite capable of killing in 20 to 30 minutes. However, moderate and controlled exercise is of benefit – many Olympic medallists have acknowledged that they suffer from the illness, although not in its severe form. In 1982 an international symposium on 'The asthmatic child in play and sport' was held in Oslo and reported six factors designed to control the severity of EIA:

- control of exercise intensity and duration
- prolonged warm-up periods
- intervals during training
- avoidance of exercise when the air is cold and dry
- increased aerobic fitness
- the use of prescribed drugs.

The best exercise for asthmatics is swimming because it helps to improve their muscle tone and physical fitness which often tend to be below average. Swimming has been found to provoke less severe asthma than an equivalent session of cycling or running. It has also been discovered that short periods of exercise of only one to two minutes *decrease* airway obstruction. The more severe the obstruction before exercise, the greater the improvement. However, exercise continued for four to twelve minutes increases obstruction.

A child with mild asthma who is not on medication should be allowed to exercise until the first onset of symptoms and then allowed to rest. Where medication is being taken, it is better used before exercise rather than waiting for breathing difficulties to develop. Inclusion in team sports is a great encouragement to a child with asthma and many can take part successfully.

Some sufferers from EIA find that taking Intal (SCG – in a dosage advised by their doctor) just before strenuous exercise prevents the development of symptoms.

Emotion

Earlier this century one school of thought labelled asthma as a psychosomatic disorder, probably starting with childhood conflict within the family. This view has now been abandoned. Asthmatics are no more neurotic than any other group in the population.

However, it is medically accepted that emotion does play a part, particularly in childhood asthma. Additionally, asthma in any serious form is a deeply disturbing illness which can distress the sufferer and other members of the family. A severely asthmatic child can be a serious problem for an entire family, even creating psychological problems for brothers and sisters. It is easy for them to feel that the sibling gets an unfair share of parental attention and concern, particularly as the asthmatic child can appear quite well between attacks.

The child who can wheeze at will is not a common

phenomenon but certainly exists. How simple to avoid going to school or monopolise attention if the symptoms of invalidism can be invoked when the occasion is right. In *Allergies: Questions and Answers*, Dr Doris J Rapp and Dr A W Frankland comment: 'Young children will verbalise openly that if they aren't given something immediately they will wheeze and promptly proceed to carry out their threat.'

The authors' advice to parents is to try not to give in to the demands of the child – instead give asthma medication and treat the child like any other. On the other hand, sometimes the problem is that parents become anxious and over-protective of a child. Although understandable, it is a response which they should guard against.

Sometimes a child's condition can improve dramatically upon admittance to hospital, and it seems that any spell away from the family can be therapeutic. Some children benefit from attending a boarding school which caters specifically for severely asthmatic children (many asthmatics at ordinary schools receive an inadequate education because of long absences). However, there are not many such schools and none within the state educational system. The Invalid Children's Aid Association will supply a list of special schools and report that fees for asthmatic children can be met by local authorities. The authority will arrange an independent medical assessment to confirm that a special school is the best course for an individual child.

Wind and temperature variations

Hippocrates was the first to observe the precipitating effect of cold in the asthmatic. Irritable airways are a feature of the illness and they can react very quickly to a sudden change in the weather. Mild humid air seems to suit asthmatics better than cold dry air, but extremes of both temperature and humidity may bring on an attack.

Sometimes an asthmatic may seem very much better on holiday. This, of course, may have some relation to change of climate, particularly if the holiday is by the sea or in the mountains. (In Europe there are a number of spas specialising in the treatment of asthma, but none in the UK.) Equally, the relaxed air of a holiday anywhere may be responsible for the improvement. Diet and inhaled allergens are both different away from home. So many different factors are involved that it is often impossible to unravel the complexities which interact to produce an attack of asthma.

Food and drink

Some patients find that certain foods and drinks can produce an attack: among the many implicated are cheese, fish, nuts and fruit. Wheezing generally starts 10 to 15 minutes after the food or drink has been swallowed. This is one of the more unusual manifestations of food allergy (see Chapter 8).

It is important for an asthmatic to avoid very heavy meals which result in an overfilled stomach pushing up against the diaphragm. This can result in an attack because the chest is constricted. Since asthma attacks often occur at night, it is advisable for the same reason to avoid meals just before going to bed.

It is also important, particularly for an asthmatic child, not to become overweight because this puts an extra burden upon the lungs.

A new allergy test which detects delayed reactions to food has been developed at the Hammersmith Hospital with the help of a grant from the Asthma Research Council. It employs histamine, one of the chemicals known to narrow the airways in allergic reaction, to provoke deliberate reactions in the food-sensitive children taking part in the trials.

Dr Nicola Wilson, honorary clinical lecturer at the Hospital, found that histamine provocation after eating foods such as nuts and chocolate can pick up an allergy missed by simple peak flow readings. This is because the reaction often occurs one or even two hours after the food is eaten and the link is difficult to establish. The test first measured the concentration of histamine needed to cause a 20 per cent reduction in peak flow. This was done both before and after challenge with food. A fall in the concentration of histamine needed to reduce peak flow *after* the food was eaten indicated food allergy.

Dr Wilson was able to demonstrate that some foods caused delayed asthmatic symptoms, and those most likely to do so were cola, ice cream and chips. She is now trying to discover what immune mechanism is responsible for the delayed reaction.

Autonomic nervous system

A body function believed to be involved to an important degree in asthma is the autonomic nervous system. This is responsible for involuntary or automatic processes, such as the regulation of muscle activity in the heart, bladder, bowels and lungs. The autonomic system has two parts:

- the sympathetic nerves, which act as an accelerator, preparing the body for 'fight or flight' by quickening the pulse and dilating the airways of the lungs
- the parasympathetic system, which acts as a brake and relaxant, carrying out digestive and restorative functions.

It is well appreciated that the asthmatic has irritable airways which contract more readily than average; one hypothesis to help explain this is that the asthmatic suffers from a disturbed autonomic nervous system, affecting the bronchial muscle.

If this is the case, it could explain why some atopic people get hay fever and others suffer from asthma, but allergists cannot yet explain why one individual suffers from one allergic disease while another – who may be of the same family – has an entirely different set of symptoms.

Other lung diseases

There are a number of occupational lung diseases which involve the immune system but are not triggered by IgE antibodies; they fall into the group of Type III reactions (see Chapter 2). They are included here for the sake of completeness and because they are well known. Some facts about them are useful as a contrast to the typical incidence of asthma.

The best-known is probably **farmer's lung** (hypersensitivity pneumonitis). In the wetter areas of the UK this disease has been shown to affect up to eight per cent of a farming population.

The finding of the specific cause of this disease (identified by Professors Pepys and Gregory and their colleagues) opened the door to the identification of other causes. Recently, for instance, it has been shown that the same sort of disease can be caused by a wide variety of inhaled organic dusts. They fall under the general term of extrinsic allergic bronchioalveolitis. It was first observed in the eighteenth century among men who were sifting and measuring grain such as wheat or barley. It may be present in an acute or chronic form.

In the first instance, a cough, breathlessness and fever occur after an interval of 4–6 hours following exposure to the particular trigger substance. Frequent episodes involve weight loss and the patient feels ill.

In the chronic form, patients gradually develop breathlessness often over a considerable period. If the condition becomes established, irreversible obstruction to lung function occurs.

Farmers who handle hay or grain which has been stored in damp conditions are typical sufferers. Symptoms can be traced to the inhalation of the tiny spores of *Micropolyspora faeni*, a mould that develops during storage. Among the sources are mouldy hay, piles of straw, damp mouldy oats, sawdust or other waste material used for bedding on a dairy farm. It has been calculated that up to 750,000 spores a minute may be retained in the lungs.

As well as farming, a number of other jobs and even hobbies present a risk. Other forms of the disease are:

- **bird fancier's disease** people who keep pigeons are at risk from inhaling the bird's dust; even building workers are warned that it can be contracted from working in the vicinity of pigeon droppings

- **malt worker's disease** caused by malt and barley dusts present in breweries
- **bagassosis** caused by mouldy sugar cane
- **mushroom worker's disease** caused by mushroom compost.

Left unrecognised with continual exposure to the allergen, these diseases can be fatal. In a study in England involving 200 patients with farmer's lung – diagnosed between 1939 and 1975 – there were four deaths and severe disability was present in approximately one-third of the sufferers. The allergen must be avoided by perhaps abandoning a hobby or installing air-conditioning.

As yet no effective mask has been devised which will prevent the inhalation of organic material. Conditions can sometimes be altered so that the trigger substance is no longer present – this has been done in the case of bagassosis. Steroids may help some patients.

Case history *In 1985 Clinical Allergy published the case history of a 46-year-old woman who developed severe reactions, including asthma, after sexual intercourse with her husband. She proved to be one of a number of cases of allergy to seminal fluid.*

She first developed asthma in 1968, four months after her fourth pregnancy. She was admitted to hospital where the precipitating factors were found to be exertion, exposure to dust or coke fumes and respiratory infection. She was discharged a week later after a course of antibiotics and bronchodilators.

The following year she developed her first attack of asthma – accompanied by urticaria and angioedema (see Chapter 7) – as a result of intercourse. She was perfectly well for two hours after making love. Then she developed a blotchy rash on her abdomen and chest which spread all over her body within an hour. Her eyes, lips and tongue were swollen as well as her face, and a cough developed with tightness in her chest and wheezing. The symptoms increased in severity over the next two hours.

An emergency injection of adrenaline brought improvement within the next 24 hours. The rash and swelling cleared up within three days. In all, she experienced four such devastating incidents after intercourse. When her husband wore a condom she was free of symptoms.

Seen in 1970, she was given skin tests to all common allergens and foods but neither she nor her husband would agree for her to be tested with his semen. Instead, her husband had a vasectomy in an attempt to prevent her distressing reaction. It did not do so.

In 1972 and 1973 she gave strongly positive responses to a skin test with her husband's seminal plasma. Subsequently she had a course of desensitisation carried out with a preparation of her husband's semen. Seen again in 1976, she reported that she could have unprotected intercourse without adverse effects.

Case history *Although it is the tendency to develop atopic illnesses rather than a specific disorder which is inherited, asthma often affects more than one member of a family. The family case history of Professor Charles Fletcher, formerly a chest physician at the Hammersmith Hospital, illustrates this effectively as well as demonstrating how much the treatment of allergies has improved in the last fifty years.*

Professor Fletcher's wife developed severe asthma when she was four in 1917. The useless treatments she suffered during her childhood included linseed poultices on her chest and a barrage of alternate buckets of hot and cold sea water thrown over her.

'Potter's asthma cure' contained atropine and helped a little but was unpleasant to inhale. Ephedrine also helped but made her feel shaky and ill. By the time she was 23, inhalers had been developed which produced a fine spray of medication which could be taken by mouth direct to the lungs. These gave relief except when she had chest infections. Then inhalers fell into disfavour because of an increase in deaths from asthma (see Bronchodilators earlier in this chapter).

With a move from the country to London her asthma improved. About this time steroid treatment became available for the first time and Mrs Fletcher took oral steroids for five years, but at a cost of thinning of the skin. A great advance was made when it became possible to inhale modified steroids as sprays. Used regularly, these controlled the asthma without being absorbed into the system.

When her asthma worsened, due to an attack of flu, for example, she resumed the regime of oral steroids for anything from two days to one month until her condition improved. Despite the everyday use of steroid sprays, she had one or two severe sudden attacks. In these instances, she had to resort to extra medication in high doses. One fine summer's day in Scotland the sudden descent of mist provoked such a severe attack that there was no response to emergency medication. Taking refuge in a car with the heater turned on finally brought the asthma under control.

The Fletchers' son, now in his 40s, suffered eczema in infancy and became wheezy at five, especially as the result of exercise. At boarding school the resident physiotherapist claimed that 50 per cent of the boys aged 13–18 lost their asthma as a result of breathing exercises. About the same proportion would have grown out of it anyway, as he did. Now he only has mild asthma well controlled by sodium cromoglycate (Intal).

His elder sister never had asthma but developed severe hay fever – now well controlled with a steroid nasal spray.

His younger sister was less lucky. She had eczema as a baby and asthma started at four. She loved country life but was highly sensitive to horses and dogs. Severe wheezing at night was prevented by taking a dose of an oral steroid at night between the ages of eight and sixteen when her asthma became milder. She was also allergic to all shellfish and once lost consciousness in Paris after eating soup containing traces of it. The rapid arrival of a doctor with an injection of cortisone followed by an ambulance with an oxygen cylinder led to a quick recovery. She was then five months pregnant and her child – now aged seven – has developed no allergic problems. Her mother now takes a portable oxygen cylinder, as well as medication, when she travels abroad.

6

Seasonal and perennial rhinitis – hay fever

Hay fever, a wretched and debilitating condition, is probably the most common allergic disease – one sufferer in ten of the population is a conservative estimate – and it is certainly the best publicised. It affects the upper respiratory tract, the nose and the eyes, but unlike asthma does not involve the lungs. For a minority, hay fever and asthma are inter-related but have to be treated separately. About five per cent of children with hay fever eventually develop asthma.

Rhinitis (from Greek 'rhis': nose; 'itis': inflammation) is either **seasonal**, caused by pollens or moulds, or **perennial** (all the year round), often caused by house dust or animals. Both types are more common among boys and the peak incidence occurs in early adolescence. Many sufferers carry the condition into adult life.

The onset of hay fever seldom occurs before the age of five but babies who snuffle continually and cannot suck with ease because they are breathing through their mouths may well be showing early signs of hay fever. In one study of 100 toddlers reported in *The Practitioner* in 1968, more than 70 diagnosed as suffering from 'recurrent colds' were in fact subject to episodes of allergic rhinitis.

Young children with hay fever often develop a typical face which is easy to recognise. They habitually breathe through the mouth and have dark circles under their eyes which have come to be known as 'allergic shiners'. Many develop the habit of rubbing their itching noses, often upwards towards the forehead, which causes a typical wrinkle to form across the bridge of the nose.

Seasonal rhinitis

Seasonal rhinitis in susceptible people is caused by breathing in pollens or spores released into the air by trees, grasses and moulds. Pollen is the botanical equivalent of sperm – it has to reach the female organ of the plant, the pistil, for seed to be formed. Trees, grasses and cereal crops all rely on vast amounts of pollens being carried by the air in order to reach their destination. Pollens can be swept hundreds of miles in the upper atmosphere, particularly in the continental climate conditions experienced in the USA. In general, brightly coloured flowers do not provoke hay fever symptoms because they tend to have heavy, sticky pollen and rely on insects to carry out pollination.

In the UK **tree pollination** begins as early as February or March with the alder and the elm. Pollination of a given species takes place later the further north the region. The oak pollinates in April and May in the UK but in June in Scandinavia. When the weather is cold for the season, pollination may be delayed.

Weather is an important factor where both pollination and sporulation (the dispersal of fungal spores) are concerned. Rainy and windless days are best for hay fever sufferers because pollens are literally washed out of the air. The return of warm, dry and windy conditions always sees a rise in the pollen count.

The **pollen count** published in newspapers during the summer months is widely believed to be for the benefit only of hay fever sufferers, but it is equally relevant to asthmatics who are pollen-sensitive and whose symptoms are potentially more dangerous. The method of taking a daily count, the responsibility of the Asthma Research Council in London, has changed little since Dr Charles Blackley flew his pioneering kites in the last century (see Chapter 1).

A sticky slide is used to collect the pollen which is then examined microscopically to take a grain count. This is finally expressed as the number of grains in a cubic metre of air. Anything over 50 is potentially troublesome for many hay fever sufferers.

Weeds are sometimes overlooked as a source of pollen. Nettles pollinate from June to August and the earlier phase can be masked by grass pollens.

Americans visiting Britain often have to be reassured that the ragweed, the main cause of seasonal rhinitis in the USA, is not found in the UK so does not present a problem. Even in the USA its distribution is uneven, not surprisingly, given the size of the country: for example, Florida's southern tip is free of ragweed yet the pollination season runs from August to November in central Florida.

Allergy to **cereal pollen** is also often forgotten. Pollination takes place well before harvest time and those most affected live or work close to cereal crops. Allergy to this group does not necessarily imply reaction to processed grain or cereals.

The most common **mould** associated with seasonal rhinitis and asthma is *Alternaria tenuis*, which is found on a variety of cultivated plants including wheat and as early blight on potatoes. The spores are dispersed in warm dry weather with a peak in August. Sometimes people who believe themselves to be allergic to strawberries are really reacting to a common grey mould, *Botrytis*, on the fruit. Moulds can thrive indoors and outside.

Some spores of moulds and fungi are present at certain times of year while others can be around all the time and so contribute to perennial hay fever. A typical example of the latter group is the mould found in piles of damp hay and may sporulate at any time of the year although most frequently in late autumn and winter. This mould is largely responsible for the condition known as 'farmers' lung' which is a Type III reaction (see Chapter 5).

Perennial rhinitis

The principal inhaled allergens involved in perennial rhinitis are **house dust,** the **dander** (skin dust) of many birds and animals and **mould spores** present the year round. In dust the mite (or its droppings) is believed to be the most potent allergen. The constituents of dust vary a great deal according to site. As well as an impressive population of mites, house dust contains fabric fragments from furnishings, particles of skin shed by family and pets, mould spores and even other species of mite apart from the well-known variety. In an office, tiny particles of paper will be prominent in the composition of dust; in a factory, concrete particles, metal dust and rust fragments.

The powdery remains of cockroaches or the tiny hairs shed from moths and butterflies can also cause inhalant problems. Allergy to cats, dogs and horses is well appreciated but it extends to hamsters and gerbils, often found in infant schools. Fish are sometimes recommended as pets for the allergic child. Unfortunately, some children prove sensitive to fish food.

There are a number of complications of chronic rhinitis, the most common being the appearance of **nasal polyps,** moist bluish-white swellings which look like a small skinned grape. People with polyps often lose their sense of smell and should see an ENT specialist. Polyps often have to be removed repeatedly by surgery. Some patients have a combination of nasal polyps, infection, asthma and aspirin sensitivity.

Symptoms and diagnosis

The allergic reaction taking place in rhinitis is better understood than the underlying mechanisms of either asthma or eczema. This is the sequence of events:

- small amounts of allergen, grass pollen for example, are inhaled and absorbed over a period of time, resulting in sensitisation

- this provokes the production of IgE antibodies, some of which cling to mast cells present in the mucosal lining of the nose
- when the same allergen is next breathed in, it provokes the release of histamine and other chemicals from mast cells.

A running nose and continuous sneezing – certainly potentially very dangerous for the driver of a car – are the two best-known symptoms of hay fever. There are many other uncomfortable features, which vary from individual to individual, including:

- a stuffed up nose and itching of the nose and roof of the mouth
- puffiness around the eyes – quite often the first warning signal of an attack
- accompanying conjunctivitis (see Chapter 4), especially in small children
- with acute symptoms, nasal membranes are discoloured, ranging from pale pink to bluish.

A physical examination confirming at least some of these symptoms is insufficient for a firm diagnosis. Skin tests (see Chapter 2) by prick, scratch or intradermal techniques will produce positive weal and flare reactions. IgE specific to a number of allergens can be measured by RAST. Nasal secretions are found to contain significant numbers of eosinophils, mast cells and basophils, all white blood cells active in allergy, in up to 80 per cent of sufferers. Tests for grass pollen sensitivity are usually carried out with multiple extracts because patients are rarely sensitive to only one grass.

All this information serves to confirm a diagnosis of allergy as well as indicating which antigens are implicated. Many potential allergens can be present in a work environment including plant materials such as green coffee dust, flour, cotton and wood dust.

Treatment

The diagnosis of hay fever presents few problems, and most patients can make it themselves. The treatment of hay fever is more controversial, particularly **immunotherapy** (see Chapter 2). Immunotherapy (also known as desensitisation or hyposensitisation) is used extensively for inhalant allergies in the USA and to a lesser extent in the UK.

The idea behind it is that by injecting the sufferer with quantities of pollens over a period of time, immunity to their effect will be built up. Although the discovery of IgE antibodies and of the mechanism of allergic reaction has disproved this assumption, some improvements in hay fever sufferers using the method have encouraged further research.

In 1984 *Clinical Allergy* published the results of a controlled trial of oral hyposensitisation in pollen asthma and rhinitis in children carried out in the UK. This followed a trial in Capetown, South Africa, comparing the effects of oral grass pollen vaccine with placebo (a blank sample) on a similar group of children suffering from hay fever – the results had shown a greater improvement in the vaccine group. The UK study involved 54 children suffering from hay fever, asthma or both. Oral mixed-grass pollen vaccine and a matched placebo were randomly given to the children to form two matched groups. The study failed to show a significant advantage for the therapy, either for hay fever or asthma and the conclusion was 'the vaccine has at best a small effect'.

Isolated deaths from anaphylaxis (see Chapter 9) have been reported following immunotherapy but with careful precautions it does not present major problems. In the UK more than four million injections of one allergen were given in 1980 without one reported death. Some allergen preparations are more hazardous than others: mould extracts are one example, especially where the patient is a child.

Even though minute amounts of given allergens are injected, patients are usually asked to remain in the doctor's waiting room for up to 30 minutes to ensure that no ill effects take place. The one case where the efficacy of immunotherapy is undisputed is when insect venoms are involved (see Chapter 9).

Research continues into this controversial field, particularly into improving allergen extracts. The subject of food immunotherapy is highly controversial and will remain so unless acceptable scientific evidence can be produced to support what is merely anecdotal at the present time (see also Chapter 9).

More conventional treatments for hay fever include the use of **antihistamines**. They are also known as 'histamine antagonists' and inhibit the release of histamine, the chemical mediator active in hay fever. Some cause drowsiness but recently developed versions, notably Triludan and Hismanal, reduce that side effect. If taken with aspirin (there are aspirin substitutes for those allergic to them) the combination is particularly effective.

Nose drops and sprays are sometimes useful and certain brands are available without prescription. However, some older children and adults tend to over-use them which may cause the nasal tissues to swell even more, increasing discomfort, and so should not be used for more than a few days at a time.

Sodium cromoglycate (SCG) is available for hay fever sufferers in the form of a nasal aerosol, drops and spray, Rynacrom. It can also be obtained in the form of a powder similar to Intal. However, in general, SCG is less successful in the treatment of hay fever than it is in asthma.

If hay fever is really severe, **steroids** in aerosol form are the most effective treatment. In a double-blind comparison, 16 out of 18 patients found steroid treatment effective: only 7 out of 19 patients reported similar success with SCG.

For severe rhinitis which fails to respond to other forms of treatment, steroids can be prescribed by mouth or by injection. This form of treatment is less popular for perennial rhinitis because of the possibility of side effects from prolonged use of systemic steroids.

Many sufferers from the perennial condition – some 20 or 30 per cent of the total number – do not display diagnosable allergy. These patients often claim to be very sensitive to changes in climate and strong smells: symptoms include headache and pain in the region of the sinuses. Hearing problems sometimes occur. They respond best to steroid treatment.

Chronic forms of rhinitis increase the risk of sinusitis – a viral or bacterial infection of the sinuses, the nasal cavities. This is a painful condition and requires treatment with **antibiotics.**

Avoidance of the allergen concerned is of course an important consideration. House-cleaning measures to reduce dust with its population of mites and other possible allergens are described in Chapter 5. An air-filtering system, particularly in the bedroom, may be worth considering if the hay fever is severe. When the pollen count is very high, it is wise if possible to remain indoors with the windows closed.

Case history *This case history illustrates well how although an atopic individual may suffer from one overriding disorder, in this case hay fever, he or she may also succumb to other associated allergies. It also shows the impact of severe hay fever – later associated with asthma – from childhood to middle age. Mrs D (in her fifties) vividly remembers her first attack of hay fever at the age of five when she joined in with the hay-making at her uncle's farm. Hay is not a very common source of hay fever (the original term of 'summer catarrh' would have been a better description) and it is very likely that these first symptoms were caused by grass pollen.*

Mrs D's first sensation was itching on the roof of her mouth – and this continued to be the earliest warning of an attack throughout her life. After returning home to London, it was not long before she suffered further attacks. Her eyes were particularly severely affected, becoming so swollen that they were almost closed. A visit to a doctor brought little more than the suggestion that she should wear dark glasses and the comment that she was probably allergic to a few things.

From the age of seven to twelve, Mrs D suffered unmitigated misery from March until September every year. Neither her mother nor her teachers were particularly sympathetic. Quite often her eyes were so swollen that she could hardly see the blackboard and all her constant sneezes provoked were cries to be quiet from her schoolmates.

She felt so desperate at 12 that she visited the family doctor on her own. He suggested that she rest in a darkened room with cold compresses on her eyes. At 17 she was blind for two weeks when her eyes became completely closed. For the first time Mrs D was referred to an ENT specialist and skin-tested for allergies. She proved positive to all 28 substances used and her arm became so swollen that she had to wear a sling for three days. She remembers the consultant reciting the litany of reactions – all positive – 'early trees, late trees, early grass, late grass . . .'

Three years earlier at 14 she had developed asthma, wheezing severely at night so that she was continually wakeful and had to prop herself up with pillows in order to ease her breathing. Over the years she received a variety of medications – Piriton tablets for hay fever, Ventolin tablets and an Intal inhaler for asthma proving the most useful.

Her life was dogged by associated infections. She had pneumonia three times and acute tonsillitis with the formation of an abscess (sometimes known as quinsy) twice. She had one other curious symptom. If a dog or cat put its nose on her bare leg, it provoked an attack of urticaria (see page 119). She had no inhalant problems with animals.

As the years passed, Mrs D learned to cope with her very considerable disabilities with courage. She mastered the ability to control her breathing with particular emphasis on breathing out which she found very helpful during an attack of asthma. As she became older, her season of illness shortened to the three months from July to September (remission of allergies often occurs in this way).

The summer of 1984 proved to be almost trouble-free for the first time since her childhood because she was prescribed a new antihistamine, terfenadine (Triludan). (This drug represents a very considerable advance on previous antihistamine therapy because it produces hardly any of the sleepiness associated with previous tablets.)

On two occasions in her life, Mrs D developed potentially serious anaphylactic reactions to substances swallowed. The first

113

instance involved a manufactured breakfast sausage stocked in the family's shop. She had eaten it for many years without any reaction until a delivery man commented that the formula had been improved.

Mrs D cut a slice and slipped half of it into her mouth. Almost immediately she suffered frightening symptoms. She felt sick, faint and very ill. Her doctor gave her an emergency injection (probably antihistamine or adrenaline) and told her to sleep it off. He commented that had she eaten the whole slice of sausage, she could have died. Mrs D decided that they would no longer stock the sausage concerned and told customers the reason. It seems possible that – in altering the formula – the manufacturer had included an extra ingredient or additive, possibly a colouring, to which Mrs D reacted violently.

She experienced a second similar reaction when she started taking tablets for hay fever one season. Such reactions have been noted and very often it is due to the colouring agent used in the coating. The manufacturer may have made an alteration to the tablet which was responsible for Mrs D's reaction, or she may have developed a sensitivity to an additive which had always been present in the tablet. (Manufacturers are now tending to reduce colouring agents in pills for this sort of reason.)

7

Urticaria and angioedema

Although urticaria and angioedema are twin conditions and generally treated as such, there is sufficient variation in symptoms for one to be distinguished easily from the other. Urticaria, often called nettle rash or hives, is extremely itchy and – as with eczema – made worse by scratching. Angioedema does not itch but is often more disfiguring. Both conditions can occur in people who appear to have no other allergies.

Urticaria is extremely common and although often caused by allergy may be provoked by many other different factors. The rash resembles a weal and flare Type I reaction – indeed this is the response which produces positive results in skin testing. The centre of the weal is pale with a surrounding red flare which looks very like a nettle sting. The eruptions involve only superficial areas of the skin. They present one of the classic symptoms following the sequence of allergic reaction – as the small blood vessels in the skin get larger, fluid escapes from them and it is this that causes the swelling and red flare. The itching is due to the release of histamine.

In contrast, angioedema takes place in deeper levels of the skin and typically affects the face, particularly the lips, tongue and the area around the eye. Hands and feet may also be involved. The swelling is more severe than in urticaria. If angioedema occurs in the throat, after taking an aspirin tablet for example, it can prove fatal.

Urticaria can be mild and transitory and it is estimated that around 20 per cent of the population suffer an attack at some time during their lives. Although it can occur at any age, typical onset is at adolescence with peak incidence occurring in young adults. The observed pattern is:

- 50 per cent of sufferers have urticaria and angioedema
- 40 per cent have urticaria alone
- 10 per cent have angioedema alone.

In general, it is easier to trace the source of these twin disorders when the condition is acute rather than chronic, when it becomes difficult, very often impossible. A diary relating to the few hours before the onset of an attack can greatly help the diagnosis. If the condition is serious, a doctor must be involved in any attempt to confirm a suspected allergen, as the risk of anaphylaxis may be present.

When urticaria/angioedema is caused by a traceable allergen, avoidance is the course always advised. If the source of a chronic condition cannot be identified, antihistamines or drugs of the theophylline type, sometimes in combination with an antihistamine, are wholly successful in treating the condition. Avoidance of aspirin and food additives can sometimes help a patient. A diet of only fresh food, eliminating dyes, benzoates, salicylates and yeasts, may be recommended.

Children prone to suffer these conditions are often found to be allergic to milk and eggs but tend to outgrow the allergy and so lose their symptoms. Allergies to other foods are sometimes more persistent, however, cod and nuts being two examples.

Urticaria

At its worst, urticaria is a disfiguring and distressingly uncomfortable complaint. The rash varies a great deal and can appear anywhere on the body. The welts typically develop in groups and can be quite small – one or two millimetres across – or sometimes many centimetres in diameter. In this case the condition is called giant urticaria.

The welts appear suddenly and seldom last longer than 24 to 48 hours. Recurrent attacks lasting less than one month are regarded as acute but outbreaks that persist longer are looked on as a chronic condition. Some allergists have observed that the welts can be evident in the late afternoon or early evening and absent at other times of the day, but are unable to account for this.

The word 'exogenous' as applied to atopic eczema is also used for urticaria caused by allergy. This form is believed to be responsible for most acute cases but does not figure to the same extent when the condition is chronic.

As in other atopic diseases, food, drugs and, rarely, inhaled and contact allergens trigger mast cells to release histamine and other chemicals when they combine with specific IgE antibodies (see Chapter 2).

Causes

Many foods can be responsible for acute attacks of urticaria, the most often implicated being shellfish, fish, nuts, peanuts (which belong to the pulse family) and eggs. **Food additives** suspected include tartrazine and other azo dyes, benzoates (used as preservatives in manufactured foods) and salicylates. The last may be present in a very wide range of items including antiseptics, toothpaste, perfumed candles, perfume, ice-cream, cakes, sweets, soft drinks, jelly and jams. Salicylates are also present naturally in many fruits, plants and trees, for instance the willow, which belongs to the *Salicaceae* family and in past centuries was used for infusions to cure headaches. **Aspirin**, introduced at the beginning of this century, is a synthetic acetylsalicylic acid, related to salicylates. Patients who are aspirin-sensitive – urticaria is a common reaction – may also be affected by salicylates, and tartrazine and other azo dyes.

Peanuts have been mentioned as another common allergen which can cause urticaria and angioedema. In 1985 *Clinical Allergy* published the results of a study of reaction to peanuts in 104 children carried out at the Royal

Alexandra Hospital for Children in Sydney, Australia. All the children were skin-tested with four peanut preparations as well as three well-known inhalant allergens – house-dust mite, cat fur and rye grass.

The results of the tests showed that:

- 60 children reacted to one or more of the inhalant allergens
- of these, 41 reacted to one or more of the peanut preparations
- 8 children had immediate symptoms on eating peanuts, suffering urticaria and/or angioedema; they all had positive results to skin tests with peanut preparations.

The medical team later identified 12 children with a history of immediate reactions to peanuts or peanut products. They ranged in age from 5 months to 14 years. In all cases symptoms of urticaria and/or angioedema were reported within minutes of eating peanuts. In addition:

- 11 of the 12 had a history of wheezing, although in only one case was the wheeze part of the immediate reaction
- 7 of the 12 also reacted to egg with urticaria and/or angioedema.

Nine of this group of children were under four. In a subsequent trial, when 300 children were skin-tested with peanut allergen, clinical symptoms were present in only one child who was over six. The research team concluded that sensitisation to peanuts may be particularly likely to occur in early childhood.

In another review of 300 patients who developed urticaria following food, it was possible to identify how many reacted to a wide spectrum of items: egg 17; strawberry 16; citrus fruit 15; fish 15; chocolate 14; pea family 13; tomato 12; milk 11; shrimp 9; walnut 9; cashew nut 6; pork 5; wheat 5.

Drugs are very common offenders in this field of allergy (see Chapter 10). Many patients are unaware that a large number of everyday medications contain aspirin. Those who are highly aspirin-sensitive may also react to other pain-killers and should always check with the pharmacist before buying a pain-killer. Besides aspirin (which can trigger many differing reactions in the atopic patient), penicillin is the best known but many other antibiotics can cause urticaria/angioedema, including cough mixtures, the contraceptive pill, sedatives, tranquillisers, tonics (quinine) and diuretics (water pills).

Inhaled moulds are the most frequent cause of urticaria. In the USA many patients report the symptoms as a result of inhaling moulds when cutting grass. One young farmer developed the condition in a severe form when he was exposed to dusts in a barn, a rich source of moulds.

Contactants occasionally cause nettle rash, such as the saliva of house pets and horses, as well as certain foods, including egg and tomato. People have developed urticaria as a result of sitting on plastic chairs or car seats covered with synthetic fibres. Sometimes dyes may also be responsible.

Although frequently brought on by allergy, nettle rash can be triggered by many other factors. Among these are **cold, infection** (especially if it is accompanied by temperature), **heat, light** and **pressure**. For some individuals, widespread welts and severe swelling can result from a swim in cold water. In these circumstances it is possible to lose consciousness and drown. This has happened rarely to children in shallow cold pools. A more common type of urticaria develops after a warm shower. Sometimes shortness of breath and wheezing occur at the same time.

Exercise urticaria

Exercise urticaria is a recently described phenomenon. Its emergence coincided with the increased popularity of strenuous exercise, particularly jogging. A typical onset includes urticaria followed by the more severe swelling of angioedema. Anyone who has suffered from such a reaction, particularly on a hot day, should take great care in exercising vigorously, since an attack can occasionally culminate in anaphylactic shock and collapse.

Dermographism

In this condition, a weal with a flare appears where the skin has been stroked firmly. The weal appears rapidly and usually fades within 30 minutes. Some patients have been found to have increased histamine in their blood following extensive stroking. It has been estimated that about four per cent of the population suffers from this curious condition.

Some forms of urticaria display a delayed response, arising several hours after the trigger has played its part. One form can often be induced by wearing tight clothes.

Angioedema

Involving the deeper skin tissues, angioedema is not itchy, but it can be painful or cause a burning sensation. The degree of swelling is often much more marked than in urticaria and sometimes the face becomes severely distorted. The eyes can be swollen to mere slits and the lips grotesquely enlarged. When the limbs are affected, they become rigid and impossible to bend.

If the condition is severe, it can very occasionally present a crisis when the swelling affects the breathing passageway. However, if angioedema does affect the glottis (the opening at the upper end of the windpipe), a doctor should be called immediately. The condition responds to an injection of antihistamine or, if serious enough, adrenaline. Anyone who has ever suffered from this type of reaction is usually advised to wear a Medic-Alert pendant or bracelet (the address is given at the end of the book). An adrenaline syringe for self-administration is also a form of extra insurance if the person's doctor considers it advisable.

Angioedema also differs from urticaria in that inhalants

are a less common cause (and for this reason skin tests are not helpful in diagnosis), and drugs are a more common factor in angioedema (see also Chapter 10).

Serious oedema (swelling) can be triggered by a wide variety of factors quite apart from allergy and these must also be explored.

Hereditary angioedema (HAE)

This is a rare disorder which features oedema of the skin, respiratory and gastro-intestinal tracts. It does not involve any form of allergic reaction, but is due to an inherited enzyme deficiency.

Case history *An issue of* Clinical Allergy *published in 1984 gave a case history of a 50-year-old man who suffered from both allergic urticaria and* HAE. *He had chronic urticarial eruptions covering various areas of his body. Interspersed with these extremely itchy attacks, swellings would appear on his face and lips which did not irritate but were painful and tender. Associated with the skin condition, he suffered frequent attacks of abdominal pain which lasted for up to 48 hours.*

In addition to the urticaria, he also had chronic hay fever and asthma for which he took sodium cromoglycate. House dust and cat dander had been identified as the allergens responsible.

The patient's father had recurrent swelling of the tongue and foot: his brother suffered from a similar condition affecting his tongue and penis. The patient had two children: a son, aged 21, suffered from chronic hay fever and recurrent abdominal pain for which he had had a number of operations without any abnormality being found. The daughter, two years younger, also had hay fever and suffered two attacks of angioedema affecting the lips. She had two periods of surgical observation for severe colicky pain in the abdomen, the symptoms finally settling down within three days. The pain was thought to have been caused by intestinal angioedema.

Positive results to RASTs *indicated that the patient's urticaria could have been due to food allergy. For this condition he was treated with an elimination diet alone. The itchy urticaria disappeared but could be provoked by dairy produce and rice. The* diet did not affect the frequency or severity of his attacks of angioedema.

For the latter condition, he was treated with danazol, a proven effective drug for HAE. This cured both the angioedema and the abdominal pain. He was later switched to another, much cheaper, type of medication. He remained symptom-free on this regime which treated two conditions – normally linked but quite separate in this case – with different forms of treatment.

8

Allergy to food: new theories

There is no controversy in medicine today that allergic reaction to food can produce frightening and violent symptoms. One type of food allergy is totally accepted by the medical world. This is immediate Type I reaction occurring in atopic people who usually suffer from other disorders also mediated by IgE (see Chapter 2). The response – vomiting, urticaria or angioedema, for example – occurs suddenly and violently soon after the food has been eaten and patients quickly learn to avoid it.

Serious reactions can occur if the food is eaten by mistake as an ingredient of a dish which hides its identity. One outstanding aspect of this type of reaction is that it can occur in response to the most minute quantity of the trigger food.

Earlier chapters have explained how children may be especially vulnerable to allergens contained in such every-day foods as milk, bread and eggs and that they may respond by developing eczema and/or asthma. There is wide acceptance that although the illnesses may not be caused by the food allergens alone, they are a contributory factor.

Gastro-intestinal allergies
Babies Gastro-intestinal symptoms are most likely to be caused by allergy where there is a family history of atopic disorders. In a study in the USA, one in three of children who had colic as babies developed asthma between the ages of six and ten, and asthmatic parents were found to have colicky babies more frequently than parents without atopic disorders.

In another investigation of 65 children with allergies aged 10 and under, 31 were found to have had a history of gastro-intestinal disturbances as babies.

Many parents are only too familiar with the symptoms of colic. Typically, an attack occurs suddenly and very often in the evening. It is clear from the prolonged and loud crying and the way the legs are drawn up that the baby has a bad stomach ache. 'Three month colic' (which can easily last six months) is not unusual in a baby who is not and never will be allergic. However, if the symptoms persist and there is reason to suppose that the baby may be at risk, allergy may well be involved.

If the symptoms are long-lasting – even if intermittent – the offending substance is likely to be cow's milk or cereal which the mother takes every day.

In *The Allergic Child* edited by Frederic Speer, MD, there is even evidence of one symptom that can occur before birth. In a study of 21 atopic women who reported foetal hiccoughs, it was possible to provoke the symptom by feeding substances to which they were allergic. Atopic disorders developed in their babies early in their lives.

Most children who develop food allergies have symptoms in infancy – 79 per cent of one group studied had developed reactions before they were one year old. The principal suspect was cow's milk and most studies concentrated on it. The difficulties were immense because milk contains several allergens.

An increase in IgE antibodies was shown in the mucosal lining of the small intestine after milk challenge in a child known to be atopic. Specialists believe that it is possible that milk allergen combines with IgE fixed to mast cells in the gut to provoke the release of chemicals in a Type I reaction (see Chapter 2).

Case history *In one family, a mother breastfeeding a colicky baby (who was also receiving cow's milk supplement) decided to eliminate all dairy products from the family diet to save doing two lots of cooking. As a result, the baby stopped screaming and* *his diarrhoea improved. His older siblings, aged eight and six, amazed a specialist who had been treating them for recurrent tonsillitis and otitis media. The conditions improved so greatly that scheduled operations were cancelled. That spring the family did not suffer usual bouts of hay fever and the children kept free of colds. At nineteen months the baby was again given milk with morning cereal and severe diarrhoea followed.*

There is no reliable laboratory test for cow's milk allergy. The following criteria are often employed:

- symptoms subside after elimination of milk from diet
- symptoms recur within 48 hours of re-introduction of milk
- this sequence is reproduced three times.

However, there are many instances when it is impossible to employ this system. For example, some children take more than 48 hours to relapse after the re-introduction of milk. (This usually occurs only when a food has been omitted from the diet for a long time and a degree of tolerance has built up.) In others the reaction is too severe to justify repeating the challenge.

When gastro-intestinal allergy is suspected in a toddler, substances other than food must be considered, including:

- aspirin or other drugs
- food preservatives such as benzoates
- flavour enhancers: monosodium glutamate, for example, which is used widely in Chinese cooking and is present in much tinned food
- artificial colours such as tartrazine.

Older children A recent study (albeit a pilot one) of twelve children aged between five and fifteen, all suffering from stomach symptoms, was reported in *Clinical Allergy* in 1984. They all had a history of abdominal pain with nausea and sometimes vomiting, and in each case there was a family history of classical migraine. Four of the children had eczema and one hay fever.

The whole group was told to follow a diet excluding eggs, dairy produce and chocolate. Where there was a previous history indicating allergy, tea, coffee and citrus fruits were also excluded. As a result of this regime, ten of the twelve experienced an improvement in symptoms, some becoming completely free of them.

Only four of the children had raised IgE levels, three associated with eczema and one with hay fever. As well as measuring total IgE level, RAST assays (see Chapter 2) were carried out to identify specific antibodies against egg white, wheat, milk, orange, yeast and cocoa.

Adults In adulthood, many people suffer indigestion with varying degrees of severity and discomfort. Very often these conditions are difficult to diagnose and treat. It is now considered that allergy may play a part in some at least of them.

Around 50 per cent of patients attending gastroenterology outpatient clinics have 'irritable bowel syndrome'. The symptoms are pain, diarrhoea and constipation.

In one study two-thirds of the patients improved on elimination diets. Of 205 patients involved, 141 were able to identify specific foods responsible for their symptoms. Foods most frequently named were wheat, dairy products and corn (maize and its many products). Other foods which affected some patients were tea, coffee, eggs, onions, potatoes and citrus fruit. The mechanism involved was not identified as allergy by any of the tests conducted.

Allergy may also play a part in the illness of some patients with chronic gastritis (inflammation of the lining of the stomach).

The clinical ecologists

Food is an emotive, often obsessional, subject in the modern world. Confusion and controversy cloud the issues – often because words are not used precisely and mean different things to different people – and it is easy to fall into the trap of regarding all ill-effects from food as allergies.

True food allergy is confined to immunological reactions. Other adverse reactions to food include:

- psychological aversion (straightforward dislike), detectable because symptoms do not occur when the food is given in unrecognisable form
- lack of important enzymes in the intestine – this affects digestion of specific food, milk for example, a condition sometimes called 'idiosyncrasy'
- reactions to substances in food which have a pharmacological effect, for example histamine in mackerel and sardines, tyramine in certain cheeses and caffeine in tea and coffee
- response to histamine released directly by certain foods, strawberries and tomatoes, for example.

But the word allergy is also being widely used now for a very different reaction producing a much wider range of symptoms, from aching joints, fatigue and headaches to depression and alcoholism. This concept of 'hidden' or 'masked' allergy is explained later in the chapter. It originated with a group of doctors in the USA calling themselves 'clinical ecologists'.

Until recently, most doctors were inclined to dismiss the theories of the clinical ecologists as mumbo-jumbo without any scientific backing and supported only by anecdotal case histories. However, scientific studies have now been carried out which provide some support for a suggestion that this type of delayed adverse reaction to food may involve Type III allergic reaction (see later in the chapter).

In the UK their society has recently been renamed the British Society for Allergy and Environmental Medicine; all the members are doctors. The movement is still separated from mainstream medicine in the UK yet its influence is gaining ground. Orthodox allergists are listening to clinical ecologists and trials have been carried out.

The tenet of the clinical ecologist movement today is that

up to 30 per cent (some put it higher) of the ills taken to family doctors in the industrialised world are due to what man is doing to the environment, including effects on food, drink, water and air. The belief is that a wide variety of ailments, both mental and physical, can be cured or at least alleviated by avoidance of these hidden or 'masked' allergens.

The father of the clinical ecology movement in the USA is regarded as being Dr Theron G Randolph, an orthodox allergist by training who developed a concept of allergy that was much wider than the traditional view. In his book written with Ralph W Moss, *Allergies – Your Hidden Enemy*, Dr Randolph credited Dr Herbert J Rinkel with the first discovery of masked allergy.

Case history *When he was a medical student, Rinkel was married with a child and suffered from a shortage of funds. Assistance came from his father, a farmer, in the shape of a large number of eggs every week. The Rinkels more or less lived on eggs.*

At that time Rinkel developed the symptoms of hay fever. Since eggs are well-known allergens, it occurred to him that egg allergy might be responsible, so he drank six beaten raw eggs but failed to react in any way, and did not pursue the idea further at that stage.

Later in his career he decided to eliminate eggs from his diet to test a hypothesis that combinations of foods might be responsible for allergies. After avoiding eggs for five days, he ate a slice of cake containing them at a birthday party. Within a few minutes he became unconscious although his pulse, blood pressure and respiratory rate remained normal; he recovered quickly. Other doctors present were at a loss to explain his collapse.

Rinkel began to wonder whether, after eating a given food very regularly – then omitting it for a period of days – a violent type of reaction would result from its re-introduction. After testing a number of chronically ill patients, his findings confirming this view were published in local allergy journals.

Dr Randolph described in his book how his observations led him to break away from orthodoxy in the field of allergy. He dropped the skin prick tests favoured by his colleagues. He declared his belief that the vast preponderance of food allergy was 'masked' because it was caused by foods eaten frequently and often in large quantities. Patients found it difficult to believe that their symptoms could be due to popular foods or environmental factors such as fumes from a gas boiler because there was no obvious link between cause and effect. Dr Randolph compared sufferers to alcoholics and drug addicts because he believed that they had a hidden addiction to the foods in question.

In discussing his theory, Dr Randolph conceded that neither the term 'allergy' – used in its strictly medical sense – nor the word 'addiction' precisely fitted the condition he was describing. The common factor providing a link with addiction was that the sufferer tended to alternate between 'highs' (stimulatory reactions) and 'lows' (withdrawal symptoms).

These stimulatory levels can be regarded as the body's adapting to foods or environmental factors to which the individual is 'allergic'. When the body can no longer adapt, withdrawal reactions or 'lows' are experienced.

Both 'highs' and 'lows' are on a scale of one (mild) to four (serious). For example, a chronically tired beer drinker who is allergic to grain may experience a lift from several whiskies (plus two). He then experiences a delayed hangover (minus three) before returning to his accustomed state of fatigue (minus two).

Critics of the clinical ecology movement have commonly dismissed the results of its practitioners as principally anecdotal. Certainly their literature abounds in case histories.

Case history *One case study included in Dr Randolph's book concerned an attractive woman in her thirties who – despite a happy marriage and rewarding job – was contemplating suicide. She had a history of asthma and stomach problems, diagnosed as viral infections, as a child.*

She did well at college although later admitted that a gradual malaise began to affect her. She felt a kind of euphoria in the chemistry lab. Severe headaches started to trouble her and on some days she could not concentrate. She relied on convenience foods, cola drinks, chocolates and sweets to combat these low periods. Because she became overweight she consulted a doctor who prescribed amphetamines. She stopped taking them because she felt she was becoming addicted to them.

Her marriage did not work well, mainly because of her irritability and unreasonable behaviour. She could not drive a car because she became so confused that she could not interpret traffic signals. She consulted a number of specialists including a psychiatrist.

All her symptoms worsened when she took a job which brought her into contact with industrial chemicals. She married for the second time and gave up her job. Another visit to a psychiatrist brought a renewed prescription for amphetamines. She went to consult Dr Randolph.

His practice was to make patients fast for five days, drinking only bottled water. He then introduced foods one at a time, beginning with fish as long as a patient had no allergy to it. Foods grown organically followed and reactions were noted from zero to four:

- *first degree – running nose, itching, mild rash, all transient symptoms*
- *second degree – more serious allergic reactions including stomach upsets*
- *third degree – either one severe reaction, such as inability to keep awake, or a large number of less severe symptoms; concentration or memory could be impaired*
- *fourth degree – rapid incapacitating symptoms; mania and convulsions were typical.*

Dr Randolph found that less serious reactions could be relieved by alkali salts or milk of magnesia whereas in fourth degree reactions it could be necessary to empty the gastro-intestinal tract by 'more vigorous efforts' and also administer oxygen. He also tested patients with products which had been grown commercially and 'sprayed copiously' to assess patients' susceptibility to chemicals.

With this particular depressed patient, the water fast first *accentuated her symptoms but after a few days she felt much better. She reacted to most of the foods she was given, particularly beef. She also proved to be highly susceptible to chemicals so had the gas heater removed from her home. Although much more cheerful and able to lead a normal life, she still became irritable in shops that proved to be heated by gas. Understanding of her food and chemical problem enabled her to lose symptoms which disrupted her earlier life.*

In the UK one of the first proponents of Dr Randolph's theories was Dr Richard Mackarness, a psychiatrist and author of the bestseller *Not All in the Mind*. As a psychiatrist, he was particularly interested in masked allergy in relation to mood changes.

Case history *One patient who had suffered from nasal congestion came to him several years later reporting that although that symptom was less troublesome, she had begun to suffer from lack of confidence, inability to concentrate and panic attacks. In her case, the major offenders proved to be wheat, Indian tea, house dust and moulds. Avoiding the food allergens and hyposensitised against the inhaled allergens, she became well again.*

More recently, Dr Vicky Rippere, a clinical psychologist, has been conducting research into the effects of masked allergy. The first chapter of her book *The Allergy Problem* is an account of her own sufferings as a result of what she calls 'intolerance to environmental factors'. In the centuries-old tradition of researchers into the ramifications of allergy, Dr Rippere was her own first patient.

Dr Rippere's book is based on studies carried out in 1979–80 with 85 individuals, 20 men and 65 women, who answered her questionnaire about adverse effects of common factors in the environment including foods, chemicals, fumes, dust, pollens, smoke, drugs and anything else encountered in their day-to-day lives. Symptoms included migraine and headaches (47 patients); respiratory symptoms (45 patients); aggression and irritability (22 patients); joint and muscle pains (19); tension (9).

Only four patients reported psychotic symptoms (delusions and hallucinations) but all four gave wheat as a source of trouble and two named cheese and ice-cream, both milk products (although much modern ice-cream makes no use of dairy produce). Three mentioned chocolate/cocoa and two sugar/confectionery.

Dr Rippere quoted the *Anatomy of Melancholy* by Robert Burton (1577–1640) which listed foods regarded as bad for those with a 'melancholic tendency'. Milk and milk products, alcohol and sugar were included just as they were by many patients in the 1978–80 survey. One surprising item of food appearing on both lists – some 350 years apart – was carrots, not generally regarded as highly allergenic.

How hidden or masked allergy is thought to work

Food allergy, whatever form the symptoms may take, starts in the gastro-intestinal tract. The immune mechanism present in 'masked' or hidden allergy is difficult to prove partly because the interval between eating the food and suffering the reaction is highly variable. For instance, one boy who was a victim of multiple allergies developed swollen lips immediately after eating eggs or nuts (angioedema), became breathless from asthma over a course of hours after eating wheat or rice and developed eczema several days after chicken.

The principal problem associated with hidden allergy is that the symptoms are so wide-ranging and sometimes only vaguely defined – including stomach upsets, a bloated feeling, headaches, pains in muscles and joints, fatigue, hyperactivity, depression and lassitude – that investigation and definition of a patient's condition, before and after diet treatment, is difficult to evaluate. This complication is accentuated in the case of children.

However, recent findings of a number of authoritative studies have provided considerable evidence of the implication of food in a variety of common ailments (see later in this chapter).

The mechanism of delayed food allergy is still poorly

understood although it has been suggested that it may belong to the Type III Gell and Coombs classification (see Chapter 2) which involves the formation of 'immune complexes'. These are amalgamations of antigen and antibody which – in the normal course of events – are a prelude to the destruction of the invader. In certain circumstances, for example if the complex becomes too large, this fails to occur.

It has been suggested that such immune complexes formed locally in the gut can be absorbed into the circulation and deposited in distant sites where they cause inflammation, for example in the brain with migraine, in skin with eczema and in the gut with irritable bowel syndrome. Although the mucosal lining of the gastro-intestinal tract normally prevents allergens breaking through to be absorbed, they may be able to escape through the lining because of an increased permeability which may be traceable to a number of sources.

One of these which has been the subject of investigation is *Candida albicans* – a micro-organism (a type of yeast) commonly present in the body. Anyone who has had thrush, either in the mouth or the vagina, knows that although innocent most of the time, *Candida* can spread and become a nuisance. If the organism spreads in the bowel it may open the way for large molecules of partially digested food to escape through the weakened mucosal lining. It may also allow immune complexes to enter the circulation.

It has been demonstrated that such immune complexes containing IgE can form following food challenge. Production of these complexes was reduced when the patient had taken sodium cromoglycate beforehand, a drug known to inhibit the release of histamine and other chemicals from mast cells.

Apart from the immunological difference between a Type I and a Type III reaction, the main differences seem to be in timing and quantity of food eaten. In a classic Type I reaction, the effects of a trigger food are immediate and can occur after only a tiny amount of the food has been eaten. A Type III reaction is delayed, and may become manifest only

133

several hours after the food has been eaten. The timing may be enormously variable. Moreover, it is common for the person to crave the food and eat a great deal of it. People with Type III hidden allergy consequently tend to find it incredible that they are allergic to a particular food.

Diagnosis

If you are suffering from a severe allergy, your doctor will probably refer you to a hospital clinic. A number of tests may be carried out to identify the causes of your problems, but the one you are most likely to come across is the **challenge or provocation test**. You will be put on an **oligoantigenic diet** – one consisting of only a few foods that rarely cause reactions: rice, gluten-free bread, lamb, fresh fruit and vegetables and olive oil forms a typical regime. You will be told to avoid drugs. After one or two weeks a small quantity of the suspected food will be reintroduced and – if your symptoms return – an allergen has been traced. Double-blind food challenge provides extra evidence.

Diets, particularly those for children, should always be carefully balanced and never undertaken without advice from a doctor or qualified dietitian. General dislike of a food and/or adverse reactions to it do not necessarily involve allergy.

The value of **skin tests** (see Chapter 2) is not universally accepted where food is concerned, if the reaction is taking place in the gut. RAST tests (also Chapter 2) which identify specific allergens are more reliable although not totally so. There are two alternative tests – PRIST and ELISA – but they are less sensitive than RAST and also expensive.

A number of other tests have been developed to aid diagnosis of food allergy. Many are controversial.

Because 'allergy' is so fashionable, private allergy clinics have sprung up in the USA in great numbers recently and the trend is already noticeable in the UK. Many of these establishments are undoubtedly doing valuable work, but some can be expensive traps for the unwary. Private clinics have been known to offer allergy tests from a sample of hair sent by post – with an enclosed cheque, of course. There is no scientific support for this practice and no test of this kind is conducted at hospital allergy clinics.

If you want to attend a private allergy clinic, check that the doctor in charge is medically qualified by looking his name up in the Medical Register at a public library.

One investigation, now discredited, is the so-called 'cyto-toxic' test for food allergies offered by organisations in the USA and the UK. These tests are covered briefly in *Allergy – immunological and clinical aspects* (1984) edited by Professor Lessof of Guy's Hospital, London. An excerpt reads: 'It has been claimed (for this test) that the white blood cells of food allergic patients die and disintegrate in the presence of food to which the patient is sensitive.' The writer goes on to comment that results of this test have been shown to fluctuate day by day. One English laboratory failed to obtain reproducible results on duplicate blood samples taken from the same patients at the same time.

In the USA, New York State has taken legal action to prevent a Californian company advertising cytotoxic testing. The company was offering to test blood samples sent by post for $350. Federal investigators sent them a sample of cow's blood and received the reply that the donor was allergic to milk, blue cheese and yoghurt. A spokesman for the New York State Health Department's immunology laboratory declared that cytotoxic tests were 'unreliable, irreproducible and invalid'.

The **sublingual food test** involves the placing of dilated solutions under the tongue by dropper; if swelling results this is regarded as an indication of allergy. The test is viewed by many allergists as ineffective.

Illnesses in which hidden allergy may play a part

Migraine
Recent evidence suggests that allergy may be an important factor in migraine affecting children, although it is clear that further studies are necessary to develop diets which may be of help in severe cases. Some researchers believe that the

symptoms of migraine are caused by temporary changes to the blood vessels in the head although they do not know why this should happen.

Not every headache is a migraine, even if the sufferer believes one to be so: specific symptoms set it apart from the normal run of headaches. A typical feature is that the pain often occurs on one side of the head (migraine is a corruption from Greek 'hemicrania': half head). Attacks are intermittent, usually accompanied by nausea and vomiting, and may continue for hours or even days. These are the symptoms of 'common migraine' which affect the majority of sufferers. If the pain is accompanied by visual disturbances – flashing lights and strange zig-zag patterns, even loss of vision – the condition is described as 'classical migraine'.

In 1983 *The Lancet* reported trials involving diet carried out by a medical team from the Institute of Child Health and the Hospital for Sick Children, Great Ormond Street, in London. The result was that 93 per cent of 88 children with severe frequent migraine recovered on oligoantigenic diets. The trigger foods were identified by reintroduction one at a time and the role of foods provoking migraine was established by a double-blind controlled trial in 40 of the children.

The group was made up of 40 boys and 48 girls aged between 3 and 16. As well as migraine

- 48 had a history of atopic disease
- 65 had a close relative with migraine
- 64 had a close relative with atopic disease.

Associated symptoms which improved included abdominal pain, behaviour disorder, fits, asthma and eczema. Those patients who suffered migraine attacks as a result of external factors, such as flashing lights or a blow to the head, no longer developed symptoms in response to provocation of this kind while they were following the diet.

The improvement in behaviour disorder was so dramatic that similar trials were carried out two years later with a group of hyperactive children (see next section).

Hyperactivity

The link between diet and hyperactivity in children, for many years and still the subject of medical controversy, is increasingly recognised as an important factor in diagnosis and treatment.

The hyperactive child presents a major problem for family, friends and school. Defined medically as hyperkinetic syndrome (from Greek 'hyper': over and 'kineo': move), symptoms often begin in babyhood. Typically, the hyperactive infant is restless, sleeps poorly and cries a great deal. Colic, eczema and allergies affecting ear, nose and throat are common.

The developing toddler seems to be in constant motion and often runs about on the toes. Behaviour is excitable and unpredictable and concentration is poor. The child also appears clumsy and has poor co-ordination between eye and hand. Some hyperactive children scratch and pick at their skin.

As they reach school age, hyperactive children's behavioural problems increase in response to the wide-ranging difficulties they experience. Aggression and disruption at home and at school are not uncommon: they may be unable to play sports because of clumsiness and lack of co-ordination. In older children, general delinquent behaviour may occur. No child presents a total range of symptoms although one of the features that many share is an overwhelming thirst. This, together with lack of concentration and general restlessness, is sometimes carried into adulthood.

The results of a major study of 76 children conducted by the Institute of Child Health and the Hospital for Sick Children, Great Ormond Street, London, were published in *The Lancet* in 1985. The children selected were severely hyperactive and so not representative of hyperactive children in general. Stringent scientific tests were carried out both in regard to the foods given and the psychological assessment of the children's behaviour before and after trials. The basic oligoantigenic diet used consisted of two meats (chicken and lamb, for example); two carbohydrates (potatoes and rice, for example); two fruits (apple and banana, for example); a green vegetable and water, calcium and vitamins. Diets were adjusted to suit an individual child and the family. Foods were selected to suit the individual taste of each child and those who did not improve were offered a second oligoantigenic diet with some different permitted items.

Excluded foods were re-introduced singly, one a week, and if symptoms did not return, the child was permitted to eat the food regularly. Foods which provoked symptoms were withdrawn at the end of the week.

Suspected foods were re-introduced in double-blind controlled tests. The two principal substances which provoked abnormal behaviour in the children were food colouring (tartrazine) and preservatives (benzoates). However, none of the 76 children reacted to these alone. (Tartrazine can turn up in unexpected places. Most people would realise it is likely to be present in commercial orange squash; fewer might suspect that it is also a common additive in packeted breadcrumbs and fish fingers.)

Forty-six foods provoked symptoms, ranging from cow's milk (which affected 35 children, the largest number reacting to one substance) to previously unsuspected items such as carrots and honey. After cow's milk, the items affecting the largest number of children were egg (20 patients), chocolate (20), orange (22) and wheat (28). Those who reacted to peanuts, a member of the pulse family, were not the same as those who reacted to other nuts.

Two children reacted to 30 foods. At the other extreme, one responded to cow's milk alone and eventually ceased to do so. Five patients reported symptoms from inhalants – one to pollen, one to perfume, two to both pollen and perfume and one to house dust.

Of the 23 children who failed to improve on their first diet, 13 accepted a modified regime and nine responded favourably to it. All nine reacted adversely to an item of the original diet when it was reintroduced.

According to the psychological assessment, return to

normal behaviour was more common among the children less seriously affected but 15 per cent of those who were severely hyperactive also improved.

Treated with an oligoantigenic diet, 62 of the children improved, 21 of them attaining a normal pattern of behaviour. A significant feature of the study was that other symptoms – abdominal pain and headaches, for example – also improved. After more than a year on their diets, five children discovered that they no longer had symptoms from some former trigger foods. Thirteen children who suffered from fits were cured by the diet. One relapsed when the diet was broken and a further three had fits again with a fever. Among the 14 whose behaviour did not improve, headaches disappeared in four out of nine and abdominal symptoms in four out of ten.

Food allergy was proposed as the most likely cause of the children's symptoms in the 1985 study but it was suggested that other factors could also be involved. It is noteworthy that 32 of the 76 children had suffered from eczema, asthma or hay fever. Fifty-two had a close relative who suffered from an atopic disorder.

Parents of hyperactive children should seek advice from their GP. They might also like to contact **The Hyperactive Children's Support Group,** which was founded in 1977 by Mrs Sally Bunday and her mother; it now has branches all over the country. Mrs Bunday's determination to help others grew out of her frustration in coping with her own hyperactive son and the difficulty she found in obtaining help for him from the medical profession.

The HACSG believes that many factors may contribute to hyperactivity, such as:

- nutritional deficiencies
- high body levels of toxic metals, lead or aluminium for example, due to atmospheric pollution
- poor pre-natal diet.

However, on the evidence of the trials reported in *The Lancet*, it is clear that diet – very probably followed by allergic reaction – is a major factor which cannot be ignored. Further work is clearly necessary in order to confirm the findings and – in particular – to simplify diets for children to eat at home. Medical and dietetic staff at the trials required training to administer the diet 'which is complicated and – unsupervised – potentially dangerous'. It was also expensive and disruptive to family and social life.

Tension-fatigue syndrome

One of the pioneers of the clinical ecology movement was an American allergist, Dr Albert G Rowe, who began work in the 1920s making many early observations which inspired his successors. For example, in 1930 Dr Rowe published a description of fatigue resulting from food allergy which he called 'allergic toxaemia' (poisoning). Today this is recognised as 'tension fatigue syndrome'.

Many patients with allergies are restless, irritable and easily tired. In some cases, of course, the uncomfortable and distressing symptoms of the allergy are quite sufficient to produce these side effects.

However it is now recognised that tension and fatigue are the main symptoms in some patients and they represent a primary allergic disorder. The syndrome may display a very wide range of behavioural disorders. Some patients find it difficult to relax: they are restless, fidgety and often clumsy and poorly coordinated. They frequently find it difficult to sleep and are unusually sensitive to temperature changes, smoke, traffic and paint fumes, noise and even the discomfort of rough clothing.

Allergic fatigue is not an ordinary sensation of being tired: it is a troublesome weariness and exhaustion. Aching muscles are a common complaint of an allergic adult and it is possible that some 'growing pains' of childhood have a similar origin.

Sometimes listlessness and anxiety may impair the ability to think clearly. Such a patient may become upset and confused. The common causes of these symptoms are inhalant and food allergens. Pollens and moulds are important in the first group while the most troublesome foods include milk, chocolate, cola and corn.

These patients do not respond to treatment with sedatives and tranquillisers. If allergens can be identified, avoidance wherever possible is the rule. However, if that proves impractical, at least the patient can learn to live with the symptoms in the knowledge that they are a recognised form of allergic reaction and not just a neurotic whim.

Kidney disease

All four types of allergic reaction classified by Gell and Coombs (see Chapter 2) may be present in kidney disease, although the most common is Type III. Very occasionally Type I immediate reaction can be present. In one group of 15 patients (11 of them male), all but one had some atopic disease, hay fever and asthma being the most common.

In four cases there was an improvement or cure of kidney symptoms following desensitisation to allergens identified by skin testing. In six cases where allergy to cow's milk was involved, kidney symptoms subsided when it was withdrawn and returned when cow's milk was again included in the diet.

There is some evidence that Type I reaction is also involved in a kidney condition associated with infections such as mumps and measles. This condition also occurs in drug reactions to penicillin, for example: other characteristics are a rash and fever. Increased IgE levels and higher eosinophil counts – typical of allergy – have been found in some patients.

Rheumatoid arthritis

A crippling and common complaint sometimes affecting young as well as old, inflammatory arthritis has many different forms. It is caused by inflammation of the joints and repeated attacks may result in deformity as muscles progressively stiffen. The involvement of the immune system is evident because antibodies have been found in the area of the inflammation, although arthritics only have a slight increase in IgE in their blood. Mast cells and basophils have been found at the sites of arthritic inflammation.

Studies of the role of food in rheumatoid arthritis are still in the early stages but several small-scale studies point to reduction of inflammation as a result of changing diet. Either fasting or a restricted milk and vegetarian diet have brought improvements in the short term, alleviating rather than curing.

Total allergy syndrome

Newspaper interest in patients claiming to suffer from this condition has encouraged medical investigation. The sufferers have mostly been women aged between 30 and 50 who were well until around 20 when they developed sensitivities to various foods, followed by adverse reactions to food preservatives, petrol fumes, perfumes and soaps.

Investigations of 'total allergy syndrome' have not supported the view that it is a clinical condition. Some sufferers undoubtedly have psychiatric symptoms. On the other hand, multiple allergy is a condition quite often encountered and sufferers often have to live severely restricted lives. However, as they age sensitivities often disappear and life becomes more tolerable.

Conclusion

The information presented in this chapter serves to emphasise that allergy should not be overlooked – as it often still is – in the diagnosis of a wide variety of diseases. It is not a question of seeing allergy everywhere accountable for the majority of man's ills. This view is just as unperceptive as the outright denial that allergy may be present.

Instead, it seems sensible to consider allergy as a possible option in diagnosis, particularly if the patient suffers from allergies or has an atopic family background.

9

Anaphylaxis and allergy to insects

Anaphylaxis is the most severe form of allergic reaction. It is a systemic reaction – in other words, it involves the whole body. Someone suffering from anaphylaxis in its severe form may complain of feeling very ill, sometimes with a sensation of impending death. There may be a feeling of faintness with misty vision. Following this brief period, various violent and frightening symptoms may occur:

- severe urticaria all over the body
- swelling in the throat (which can alone prove fatal)
- breathing difficulties
- nausea, vomiting and acute abdominal pain sometimes followed by diarrhoea
- a sudden drop in blood pressure
- unconsciousness.

This last state can be reached in 5 to 30 minutes after the allergen enters the body. If someone rapidly becomes unconscious, the risk of dying is considerable. Someone who becomes unconscious in 15 minutes will become so in 10 minutes on any future occasion.

Anaphylaxis can result from a number of causes:

- violent reaction following the eating of food. The items most commonly involved are nuts and shellfish (see Chapter 8)
- drug reactions (see Chapter 10)
- systemic shock as a result of skin testing or immunotherapy (very rare).

Insect stings are also sometimes responsible for anaphylactic shock. Most of the rest of this chapter is devoted to them.

Insect stings

Allergic reactions to insect stings are not uncommon. A non-allergic person can tolerate up to 500 stings from a swarm of bees. There will be flushing, pain and swelling as well as shock attributable to such a large dose of bee venom, and sometimes a feeling of faintness, but there will be no lasting effects. In contrast, in someone who is highly allergic to bee venom, a single sting can cause the most violent symptoms which can lead occasionally to rapid death. Allergists sometimes say that such an individual is 'exquisitely' sensitive. More usually, however, the person has been stung before and has reacted abnormally to these earlier sensitising stings.

It may not be easy to tell after the first sting if you are likely to suffer a more serious reaction the next time. Positive skin tests are not always found in patients who have anaphylactic reactions to stings. Of one group of 182 patients with a history of sensitivity to bee stings, only two-thirds had positive skin tests to venom.

It is possible to detect the presence of IgE specific to venom in blood serum by a RAST assay (see Chapter 2). Unfortunately, the result does not always correlate with a patient's history of response to stings, nor is it an indicator of the severity of possible future reactions. This illustrates how – even with the most sophisticated diagnostic methods available – allergic reaction retains an elusive factor.

Treatment
It is natural that anybody who has ever suffered this type of horrific reaction becomes almost pathologically afraid of being stung again. In past centuries there was little that could be done for someone dying of anaphylaxis as a result

of an insect sting. Death from sunstroke or heart failure must have been the sorts of reason entered on death certificates.

Today, an emergency injection of adrenaline is the standard treatment for anaphylaxis. A large dose of antihistamine is often effective if the symptoms are comparatively mild. An emergency kit is available in the form of a syringe containing adrenaline. If you are at severe risk, having already reacted to insect stings, your doctor may authorise the issue of a kit so that you feel more confident at the prospect of a future emergency. However, a more simple solution is to have an adrenaline atomiser of the type used by asthmatics. Two puffs taken every 5 minutes will help to reduce symptoms until medical assistance arrives.

Once the immediate crisis is over, anyone who has suffered shock may sometimes continue to have prolonged symptoms. If this is the case, steroids can be used as an effective treatment. They are useless in the immediate crisis of anaphylactic shock because they may take four to six hours to be effective.

Immunotherapy

In many instances a crisis of this magnitude can be prevented by immunotherapy (see Chapter 2) which, despite being a 'last-ditch measure' in some other instances, is regarded as particularly effective in the case of allergy to insect stings.

When first introduced, whole-insect allergenic extracts were used – in other words, not just the venom of the insect. It is now generally recognised that venom therapy is much more effective. Whole-insect therapy was also open to criticism in that it could occasionally provoke illness resembling serum sickness (see Chapter 10).

Case history *The breakthrough was made in 1974 when a team from the Johns Hopkins University School of Medicine in Baltimore, USA, used honey bee venom for the first time. They did so because a boy was obviously at serious risk of dying from a bee sting. His sister had already died from anaphylactic shock after* *being stung. The boy himself had been seriously ill on two occasions after stings, the second despite the fact that he had been receiving whole-insect injections. The father was a beekeeper and with the approach of summer the medical team reasoned that if the boy was stung again he could well die too.*

With the help of the father who collected the bee venom himself by letting his bees sting one side of a cellophane membrane and collecting the venom which came through, a course of immunotherapy using the venom was started cautiously with increasing doses of venom being given over two months. In that time the boy was injected with the equivalent of 28 bee stings. At the end of the course he could tolerate two bee stings without ill effect.

Laboratory tests during the time of treatment indicated that an increased level of IgG, the blocking antibody (see Chapter 2), was present in the boy's blood. (A later trial of 19 patients who had been treated with venom showed that only one had a subsequent reaction to a sting.)

Identification of the insect

Sensible measures can be taken to avoid insect stings and the first priority is to identify the creatures responsible, but this might not be as easy as it sounds, since people who have had frightening symptoms as a result of a sting very often cannot remember exactly what it looked like. It is best to try to do so because allergy is often confined to one insect.

All insects have bodies divided into three parts (head, thorax and abdomen). The head carries two feelers: there are three pairs of legs and usually two pairs of wings. The group includes bees, wasps, hornets, lice, beetles, ants, flies and mosquitoes.

In the UK, bees and wasps are the species most likely to be responsible for severe symptoms. There are 290 species of wasp, most of which will sting only when disturbed. Honey bees are the most numerous of their particular group and are common wherever there are flowering plants. They are not normally aggressive except when they sense that the hive is under threat. The furry bumble bee is a separate species which makes a good deal of noise but does not sting without reason.

Now that there is so much overseas travel, foreign insects can be encountered for the first time. Hornets, a giant wasp, are common in southern Europe and North Africa. They can inflict a particularly nasty sting but because they are so big and noisy it is easy to avoid them.

In the USA fire ants that were originally native to South America are now thriving. Initially, the fire ant clamps well-developed jaws on the skin and then rotates its body to inflict a number of stings. It is estimated that two and a half million people are stung by them each month and around 16 per cent undergo systemic reactions, with some deaths.

Avoiding insect stings

Most stings occur when the insect has not been seen. Typical examples are the bare-footed child stepping on a bee on the lawn or someone encountering a wasp in a washing-up bowl. Insects flying around seldom sting without provocation.

The best line of defence is avoidance and there are a number of measures which can be taken:

- do not wear brightly coloured clothes, particularly if they are flower-patterned, as these may attract insects
- avoid the use of perfume or after-shave for the same reason
- take special care when washing up – insects are attracted to sticky foods like jam
- use insect repellant, especially on a picnic
- take care when lifting the lid of the dustbin – a favourite haunt of insects
- don't flap your arms or panic if you see stinging insects – it can make them aggressive
- if you suspect that there is a wasps' nest in your home or garden (much activity can be the clue), don't try to deal with it yourself. Local authorities usually employ pest control teams who will deal with a nest quickly and effectively.

Insects and inhalant allergies

Allergic reactions to insects and other small creatures are not confined to the effects of a sting. Spiders, which belong to a separate group called arachnids, have different features from insects. They have only two body segments, four pairs of legs and no wings or feelers. The dust mite – such an important cause of inhalant allergy – is a member of this group.

Inhalant problems traceable to minute particles of dead insects in dust are not uncommon. Allergies believed to be caused by flour or cereal dusts sometimes can be traced instead to the weevils which develop during storage. Allergy to various species of cockroach has been investigated in countries as far apart as Thailand and Puerto Rico. Very occasionally, inhalant allergens can be responsible for anaphylactic reaction.

Case history *An airline pilot who suffered mild seasonal hay fever caused by grass pollen in the UK developed severe asthma on visits to Egypt. He became certain that it was due to the Nemeti fly, a type of midge, which swarmed along the banks of the Nile in summer. When skin testing for this insect became possible, it was discovered that patients in both Egypt and the Sudan had inhalant allergies – asthma or hay fever or both – traceable to the Nemeti fly.*

10

Allergy to drugs

Harmful reactions to drugs occur frequently – a doctor must often weigh the benefits of medication against known risks – but only a minority are due to true allergic response. When such is the case, the reaction may be due to either the Type I or the Type IV reaction (see Chapter 2), although the mechanisms involved may not yet be fully understood.

Type I immediate reaction is dangerous and can cause widespread urticaria, angioedema, asthma, rhinitis and anaphylactic shock. A patient known to react in this way should wear a Medic-Alert bracelet or pendant giving details of the drugs to be avoided (the address is given at the back of the book).

Type IV reaction is described on page 29.

The picture is complicated in two ways. First, pseudo-allergy – allergic-type reactions, sometimes severe (see Chapter 2) – can occur in non-atopic individuals. This means that the symptoms of allergy are present without the classic events of allergic reaction, including the formation of IgE. A typical example is the ability of the chemical compounds in some drugs to react directly with a body's mast cells and stimulate them to release histamine. (Some foods may also have this ability – egg white, strawberries and shellfish have been suggested as examples.)

Secondly, all drugs have side effects. When someone is especially susceptible to these, the term used is drug 'intolerance'. Another word sometimes employed is 'idiosyncrasy' – the same two words used with regard to harmful effects from food (see Chapter 8). In these patients, deficiency of an enzyme means that a particular drug can cause unpleasant reactions unrelated to its usual side effects, and allergy is not involved.

It is not necessary to be atopic to display allergic symptoms to drugs although highly allergic patients and those with debilitating diseases have a higher incidence of drug-induced symptoms. It seems that women are particularly prone to develop drug allergies.

Sometimes a doctor is faced with a dilemma, especially in instances where infection is known to be present: is the rash caused by the disease or by the drug treatment? Many childhood ailments involve rashes and viral infections very often produce skin symptoms in infants. The list of drugs capable of causing skin reactions is very long: as well as penicillin and other antibiotics, aspirin, local anaesthetics and insulin (see below), it includes barbiturates, codeine, ephedrine, the contraceptive pill, quinine and sulphonamides.

Penicillin and other antibiotics

The drug most widely associated with allergy is penicillin although many other antibiotics can have a similar effect.

Reactions are said to take place in two to five per cent of patients treated with penicillin. The most common manifestations of this type of allergy are eczema, angioedema and urticaria and, more rarely, exfoliative dermatitis (a severe skin disorder). Ten per cent of reactions are life-threatening.

Analysis of a number of instances where reactions have been severe, even fatal, has revealed a number of characteristic factors:

- about 75 per cent of patients dying of penicillin anaphylaxis had no previous history of allergic reactions to antibiotics
- in most fatal cases, the onset of allergic symptoms occurred within 60 minutes
- patients who experienced severe reactions outside a hospital were unconscious before medical help arrived.

The safest method of administering penicillin seems to be by mouth. In the USA an investigation revealed only six deaths from penicillin taken orally compared with between 100 and 300 fatalities reported annually as a result of antibiotic injections.

Aspirin

Aspirin is the drug most likely to cause asthma. Sensitivity to it often occurs in patients who are allergic to many foods and inhalants. Very often they also prove sensitive to other pain-killers such as ibuprofen.

Another typical patient is non-atopic, in middle age, and has taken aspirin without difficulty for many years. About 15 per cent of them prove to be sensitive to tartrazine as well (see Chapter 8). Likely reactions to aspirin and related salicylates (see Chapter 7) in this group are urticaria/angioedema, combinations of rhinitis, nasal polyps, and asthmatic bronchitis, and anaphylactic shock, sometimes fatal.

The treatment of hypersensitivity to aspirin is complete avoidance of the drug, as well as tartrazine, if it is also implicated.

Reactions resembling serum sickness

Von Pirquet first identified serum sickness early this century. Later it was discovered that the cause was the horse serum used for diphtheria immunisation. Today serum sickness (a Type III reaction – see Chapter 2) is a rarity but a number of drugs produce symptoms closely resembling the original condition. The symptoms include fever, skin eruptions and general aches and pains. The reaction subsides once the drug is discontinued. Penicillin (especially the long-lasting preparations), is one of the most likely drugs to cause this rare reaction although sulphonamides and streptomycin have also been found implicated.

Local anaesthetics

These are among the most frequently used drugs in medi-cine. Occasionally, they cause allergic reactions of varying severity. Sometimes, if a patient has a history of allergy, a precautionary skin test may be performed based on the case history and on the local anaesthetic to be used by the dentist or surgeon. A challenge test (see Chapter 2) is a useful alternative.

Reactions to radiocontrast media

These materials are a type of dye sometimes injected before X-rays are taken because they help to produce a more sharply defined image. Occasionally, a response occurs which mimics IgE reactions. If symptoms are severe, they are treated as an anaphylactic crisis with administration of antihistamine, corticosteroids or adrenaline.

The symptoms can sometimes include a drop in blood pressure, nausea, vomiting and shock. This condition can also be treated successfully with adrenaline. No pre-testing for reactions to these dyes is possible and if a contrast media study is essential, the standard practice in many hospitals is to treat the patient in advance with an antihistamine or corticosteroid.

Insulin allergy

Current insulin preparations for diabetics are highly purified but still contain minute quantities of beef and pork protein as well as other trace substances. Preparations usually contain both beef and pork but forms with just beef or just pork are available. Beef is more allergenic than pork. Diabetics who prove allergic to both preparations may be able to use a synthesised human insulin preparation.

Most patients who have been receiving insulin for two months or longer – with or without complications – make detectable antibodies against it. Forty per cent of these will give positive weal and flare skin tests.

Local skin reactions in the area the insulin injection is given occur in about half of all diabetics. They are insignificant and transitory in 95 per cent of cases. Local reactions of this type resolve in their own time and there is no need to consider changing the type of insulin injection used. However, sometimes these localised skin reactions persist or become severe. In these cases, antihistamines taken for several weeks often clear up the problem, but if this treatment fails, a change to single pork insulin may be the answer.

Patients are always warned not to discontinue insulin therapy. If they did and the treatment had to be resumed in later life, the possibility of severe systemic allergic reaction would be quite possible. They should also be warned that an increase in inflammation locally may precede systemic reactions. Although severe urticaria is the most common systemic symptom, there have been cases of anaphylactic shock. An anaphylaxis kit (syringe filled with measured dose of antihistamine or adrenaline) should be provided for the patient's own use.

11

Complementary medicine

Many people are clearly not satisfied with orthodox medicine. Every year an increasing number of people consult complementary practitioners: it is calculated that more than a million now do so, spending around £50 million in fees. These figures take no account of the very considerable sums spent in health food shops which stock ranges of herbal and homoeopathic remedies.

Despite its new status, the field remains highly controversial, mainly because its methods are untested by any scientific principles. However, the British Medical Association has set up a working party to enquire into alternative therapies under the chairmanship of Professor James Payne. As an anaesthetist, the Professor is on record as saying he finds the achievements of acupuncture (the fastest growing of the alternatives) impressive. The BMA report is scheduled for publication later this year (1986).

Many practitioners of complementary medicine refused to give evidence to the enquiry because all the members of the panel were orthodox doctors. Yet there are open-minded medical men who warn that the charge that complementary medicine is unscientific and its claims unproven could backfire. Many orthodox treatments are likewise not well understood – this is particularly true of a large number of drugs which often have serious side effects.

The Institute for Complementary Medicine prefers the term in their title to 'alternative medicine' because they believe that their practitioners can work alongside orthodox doctors to the benefit of patients. The Institute encourages research and publishes newsletters. It has established 50 information points nationwide, manned by volunteers. Advisory and education committees have been set up to provide a professional basis to encourage standards of practice and training.

The Institute represents five principal therapies of which two, osteopathy and chiropractic, may have little relationship to allergy as they deal with the structure of the body, and disorders involving muscles and bones, such as lumbago, sciatica, hip problems and headaches related to muscle contraction in the neck.

The three therapies most likely to interest a sufferer from allergies are:

- **homoeopathy** based on the principle of 'like curing like' and said to stimulate the body's natural healing power
- **acupuncture** literally 'needle insertion', practised in China for thousands of years. It is claimed to stimulate points on the body so that the body's own healing power is set in motion
- **herbal medicine** based on traditional whole plant remedies, all characterised by low toxicity, lack of both side effects and withdrawal symptoms.

Some 30,000 alternative practitioners were listed in a recent UK survey yet only 10,000 belong to professional associations. If you are considering undergoing one of these therapies, check first that the practitioner is a member of a recognised association.

Homoeopathy

Known since the time of the ancient Greeks, homoeopathy is the practice of treating like with like. This means that a medicine which produces the symptoms of a disease in large doses is said to cure it if given in very small amounts.

Homoeopathy differs from orthodox medicine in basing treatment upon the theory that symptoms are the body's

155

reaction against the illness, rather than caused by the illness, and must be stimulated rather than suppressed.

Modern theories of homoeopathy were developed by a German doctor – Samuel Hahnemann (1755–1843) – who discovered that a small dose of quinine produced the symptoms of malaria in a healthy person. Known as 'cinchona', quinine was even then a standard remedy for malaria.

Hahnemann and his followers carried out a series of systematic experiments with a wide variety of remedies, noting the symptoms produced. Patients suffering from similar complaints were then treated with the substances. Their results have been described as 'usually encouraging and often remarkable'.

They discovered that a remedy generally became more effective the more it was diluted. Hahnemann worked to establish the smallest effective dose, realising that this was the best method to avoid side effects from treatment.

The homoeopathic doctor aims at treatment of the whole person rather than prescribing for a set of symptoms. Knowledge of the person's life history forms the basis for treatment. For this reason, patients with a similar disorder may receive different remedies. Some patients find that their condition deteriorates for a few days before they experience an improvement but this is not general.

Surgery is not ruled out in cases of advanced disease but the homoeopathic practitioner believes that it can prove unnecessary if treatment is started soon enough.

Homoeopathic medicines are available under the NHS and some can be bought at health food shops. However, because treatment should ideally be tailored to the individual, it is regarded as much more satisfactory to consult a homoeopathic doctor.

Acupuncture

The first recorded success of treatment by acupuncture was made more than 2,000 years ago in China. Today, more than one million Chinese doctors practise this form of treatment, often in conjunction with diet, massage, hydro-therapy, herbalism and exercise.

The British Acupuncture Association makes it clear that other forms of treatment should be used in degenerative illnesses. However, many functional disorders (including eczema, migraine and asthma) may benefit from acupuncture alone.

The underlying belief is that dual flows of energy called Yin and Yang exist in the body as well as being expressed in the universe in day and night, hot and cold, life and death. Yin, the negative force, tends to sedate and expand; Yang, the positive force, stimulates and contracts. In the body, health is dependent upon the equilibrium of these two forces.

Together they circulate in the body along channels known as meridians – these can be detected by electronic means. There are twenty-six main circuits, each associated with a different body function or organ.

In disease, energy flows of Yin and Yang become un-balanced and often certain points in the body become pain-ful when pressed. These are associated with a condition which is developing and can enable a practitioner to diagnose oncoming illness as soon as a patient's health deteriorates.

Energy flow can be stimulated or sedated and equilibrium between Yin and Yang restored by piercing the skin at certain points. There are more than 600 of these points.

An important recent innovation has been the introduction of electro-acupuncture. For the first time this permits the taking of objective diagnostic readings which are essential to research carried out by Western science. A patient can be tested before and after treatment, also from treatment to treatment.

An experienced acupuncturist can distinguish many variations in the pulses. This will help him decide which meridians require to be balanced and which points to needle.

Needles are inserted in the skin to varying depths, according to the point and condition to be treated. The length of time they are left in place may vary from a few seconds to several minutes.

Because anyone can set up as an acupuncturist, with little training, you should find a local practitioner by consulting the British Acupuncture Association. Full members of the Association have qualified at the British College of Acupuncture as well as training in basic western medical sciences.

If an acupuncturist does not appear on the register, the Association will check a practitioner's qualifications on behalf of potential patients. Acupuncture can only be obtained on the NHS in rare cases from one of the few hospitals where it is practised. Fees charged by individual acupuncturists vary.

Herbal medicine

The National Institute of Medical Herbalists was established in 1864. Membership is by examination after completing a four-year course of training. A period of clinical practice must be completed before the final examination is taken. Qualified practitioners carry the letters MNIMH or FNIMH after their names. A copy of the register of herbalists can be obtained from the Institute by sending a large stamped addressed envelope.

Diet, exercise and life-style are all important to the herbalist who disapproves of the isolation of pure drugs which is part of medical orthodoxy. It is believed that whole plant remedies, containing many different constituents, provide more balanced and much safer remedies.

The Institute points out that herbal medicine was common to ancient civilisations and modern research has confirmed many early beliefs about the medical properties of various herbs. The National Institute has its own research department but because of lack of resources, more than 750,000 species await investigation.

The herbalist claims that plant medicines 'are characterised by their low toxicity, their lack of accumulation and side effects and by the absence of habituation and withdrawal symptoms'.

Holistic medicine

The British Holistic Medical Association was founded in 1983 by a group of doctors dedicated to an approach to health rather than any specific method of treatment. It now has several hundred doctors as members. One of the aims of the Association is to foster a different relationship between doctors and patients in the belief that disease can result from many patterns of behaviour in relation to diet, relaxation, exercise and relationships.

Holistic medicine asserts that health care should imply not only physical health but psychological, emotional and spiritual health. It believes that each individual has an ability to effect self-cure to a greater or lesser extent. The Association embraces all forms of treatment – orthodox and complementary medicine as well as self-help skills which include breathing and relaxation routines, meditation, exercise and diet.

In 1984 associate membership was offered to the lay public and a few months later the British Association for Holistic Health was launched, offering membership to practitioners from other disciplines – acupuncture for example – as well as nurses and social workers.

Many doctors already practise holistically without using the term, and a proper investigation of allergies will always draw up a case history of every aspect of a patient's life. It is the aim of the BHMA to influence medical opinion so that this wider approach to health becomes more generally accepted.

Although these are the principal disciplines of complementary medicine many other techniques may benefit an individual. For example, the practice of yoga, leading to an increased sense of relaxation and wellbeing, may help an atopic individual; hypnotism may likewise be of value.

In all instances, before embarking on a course of treatment, it is sensible to check on the qualifications of the practitioner or teacher involved by contacting the appropriate association.

Postscript

Both the understanding and treatment of allergies are expected to improve dramatically in the next ten years.

Immunology, which has been described as the science of the future, is expanding rapidly: specialists have to work hard to keep abreast of new developments. In allergy, it is clear that the full story is not yet known. Antibodies belonging to groups other than IgE may also play a significant role. Delayed responses – which do not fall into the Type I allergic classification – could contribute to many disorders, particularly where food is involved.

The theories of masked allergy to commonly eaten foods need to be subjected to rigorous scientific trials. The studies (reported in Chapter 8) on diet in children suffering from migraine and hyperactivity have pointed the way. Neither condition belongs to the classic group of atopic illnesses yet the children's health improved with changes in diet. It is noteworthy that a number of them also suffered from recognised allergies.

Because the field is so diverse, research adopts many different approaches. In Finland, Professor Matti Tolonen of the University of Helsinki has written a bestseller on the importance of vitamins and minerals. In one of his studies, atopic eczema improved in 20 children given supplements of zinc and gamma-linolenic acid (GLA). In this country, trials with evening primrose oil (Efamol) have produced promising results in eczema patients (GLA is a constituent of the oil).

Much remains to be done before reliable statistics on the

incidence of allergy can be prepared. Although the prick test is well proven, no standardised procedures exist.

Even starting to understand allergies has taken many thousands of years to achieve. Conquering them – already under way – is the next step.

Glossary

acute	temporary and severe
allergen	substance causing an allergic reaction
allergy	symptoms occurring in response to a previously encountered substance despite the fact that it is harmless; a 'malfunction' of the immune system
anaphylaxis	a severe allergic reaction which can lead to collapse, even death
angioedema	swelling in the skin and underlying tissue
antibody	a protein produced in the body in response to invading foreign materials: also called an immunoglobulin
antigen	any invading substance which provokes an immune response
antihistamine	a drug which blocks the effects of histamine, released by mast cells in the body during an allergic reaction
atopy	a hereditary tendency to Type I allergic reaction
basophil	white blood cell which releases chemicals during allergic reaction; similar but not identical to mast cell
B cells	white blood cells derived from bone marrow which are involved in production of antibodies; also called B lymphocytes

bronchodilator	drug that relaxes the smooth muscles in constricted airways; often used in acute asthma
chronic	long-lasting
corticosteroids	group of hormones produced by the adrenal cortex which play many key roles in body function, including metabolism and resistance to stress; man-made corticosteroids are used as powerful anti-inflammatory drugs in severe allergic reaction
dander	small scales from animal skin; it often acts as an allergen
desensitisation	see hyposensitisation and immunotherapy
eosinophil	white blood cell present at site of allergic reaction
gastro-intestinal tract	stomach and intestines
histamine	chemical released by mast cells considered responsible for the itching and swelling of hay fever and other allergies
hypersensitive	allergic
hyposensitisation	term used to describe immunotherapy
immunoglobulins	family of proteins to which antibodies belong
immunotherapy	injections of gradually increasing amounts of allergens known to trigger a patient's allergic response
leukotrienes	chemical mediators of allergy
lymphocyte	white blood cells of two major types, T and B, which are important in immunity and allergy

mast cell	tissue cell which contains packets of chemicals which – when released – cause the symptoms of allergy
placebo	dummy pill, blank sample drug
prostaglandins	group of fatty acids involved in many bodily functions; they constrict smooth muscle in allergic reaction
proteins	complex chemical substances made of amino acids; essential constituents of all living cells
rhinitis	inflammation of the membrane lining the nose; allergic rhinitis is hay fever
sensitise	to expose to an allergen for the first time which will provoke a response in the immune system upon subsequent encounters
sinusitis	an inflammation of the air spaces at the back of the nose
steroids	see corticosteroids
systemic	(of drug treatment) given by injection or by mouth to reach the body organs through the blood
T cells	white blood cells which are responsible for cell-mediated immunity; also called T lymphocytes
topical	(of drug treatment) applied directly on to the affected part
urticaria	skin reaction marked by swelling, redness and itching; also called nettle rash or hives (see Chapter 7)

Bibliography

* recommended reading

Adult asthma by T J H Clark, MD, BSc, FRCP (1984 Churchill Livingstone)

The allergic child edited by Frederic Speer, MD (1963 Hoeber Medical Division, Harper & Row)

Allergies by F E Graham-Bonnalie, BA, MB, BCh (Cantab), MRCS, LRCP (1970 David and Charles)

**Allergies: questions and answers* by Doris J Rapp, MD and A W Frankland, MD (1976 Heinemann Health Books)

**Allergies: your hidden enemy* by Theron G Randolph, MD and Ralph W Moss, PhD (third edition 1984 Thorsons Publishers)

**The allergy encyclopaedia* edited by the Asthma and Allergy Foundation of America and Craig T Norback (1981 Mosby Medical Library)

Allergy in children by J A Kuzemko (reprinted 1979 Pitman Medical Publishing)

Allergy – immunological and clinical aspects edited by Professor M H Lessof (1984 John Wiley & Sons)

The allergy problem by Vicky Rippere, MA, PhD, BSc, MPhil (second impression 1984 Thorsons Publishers)

Allergy therapeutics by Keith Eaton, LRCP, LRCS, LRFPS; Anne Adams, SRN, NDN; Janet Duberley, SRN, RSCN (1982 Bailliere Tindall)

**Asthma and hay fever* by Allan Knight, BSc, MD, CM, FRCP(C), FACP (reprinted 1984 Martin Dunitz)

BIBLIOGRAPHY

Asthma in childhood by A D Milner, MD, FRCP, MRCS, DCH (1984 Churchill Livingstone)

Asthma: similarities and contrasts in children and adults – report of international conference in Montreux, Switzerland (1984 Medical Education Services)

Asthma: the facts by Donald J Lane and Anthony Storr (1981 Oxford University Press)

The asthmatic child in play and sport edited by S Oseid and A M Edwards (1983 Pitman Books)

Basics of food allergy by J C Breneman, MD (1978 Charles C Thomas, USA)

* *Chemical victims* by Richard Mackarness, MB, BS, DPM (1980 Pan Books)

Clinical allergy edited by Frederic Speer, MD (1982 John Wright PSG Inc)

Clinical reactions to food edited by Professor M H Lessof (1983 John Wiley & Sons)

Current perspectives in allergy edited by Edward J Goetzl and A B Kay (1982 Churchill Livingstone)

* *Eczema and dermatitis* by Professor Rona Mackie, MD, FRCP (1983 Martin Dunitz)

Food allergy (1985 Edsall summaries for health professionals No 2)

Food for thought by Maureen Minchin (1982 Alma publications)

Footnotes on allergy by D Simon Harper (1980 Upplands Grafiska AB, Uppsala, Sweden)

The hyperactive child by Belinda Barnes and Irene Colquhoun (1984 Thorsons publications)

Immunology at a glance by J H L Playfair (third edition 1984 Blackwell Scientific Publications)

Immunology simplified by T R Bowry MB, MRCPath (Oxford University Press 1984)

Not all in the mind by Richard Mackarness, MB, BS, DPM (1976 Pan Books)

Practical allergy and immunology edited by William B Klaustermeyer, MD (1983 John Wiley & Sons Inc)

Proceedings of the first and second Fisons food allergy workshops (1980, 1983)

Stepping stones in allergy by Leon Unger, MD, FACA and M Coleman Harris, MD, FACA (1975 Craftsman Press, Minneapolis)

* *Your child with eczema* by Dr David J Atherton (William Heinemann Medical Books 1984)

Address list

Most of the following organisations ask that when writing to them for information you should enclose a large stamped addressed envelope.

Action Against Allergy
43 The Downs
London SW20 8HG
(01) 947 5082

Asthma and Allergy Treatment and Research Centre
12 Vernon Street
Derby DE1 1FT
(0332) 362461

Asthma Society and Friends of the Asthma Research Council
300 Upper Street
London N1 2XX
(01) 226 2260

British Acupuncture Association
34 Alderney Street
London SW1V 4EU
(01) 834 1012

British Holistic Medical Association
179 Gloucester Place
London NW1 6DX
(01) 262 5299

British Migraine Association
178A High Road
Byfleet
Weybridge
Surrey KT14 7ED
(093 23) 52468

Cotton On (suppliers of cotton clothing)
29 North Clifton Street
Lytham FY8 5HW
(0253) 736611

(Dead Sea salt and allied products, suppliers of:)
Finders
Freepost (no stamp needed)
Winchet Hill
Goudhurst
Cranbrook
Kent TN17 1JY
(0580) 211055

Homoeopathic Development Foundation Limited
19A Cavendish Square
Suite 1
London W1M 9AD
(01) 629 3204

Hyperactive Children's Support Group
59 Meadowside
Angmering
Littlehamptom
West Sussex BN16 4BW
(0903) 725182

Institute for Complementary
Medicine
21 Portland Place
London W1N 3AF
(01) 636 9543

Invalid Children's Aid
Association
126 Buckingham Palace Road
London SW1W 9SB
(01) 730 9891

Medic-Alert Foundation
11–13 Clifton Terrace
London N4 3JP
(01) 263 8596

National Eczema Society
Tavistock House North
Tavistock Square
London WC1H 9SR
(01) 388 4097

National Institute of Medical
Herbalists
34 Cambridge Road
London SW11 4RR
(01) 228 4417

National Society for Research
into Allergy
PO Box 45
Hinckley
Leicestershire LE10 1JY

Acknowledgements

The author would like to thank the following for their generous assistance in the research of this book:

The American Academy of
  Allergy
The Asthma and Allergy
  Foundation of America
The British Library
The British Society for Allergy
  and Clinical Immunology
The British Society for Allergy
  and Environmental Medicine
The Hospital for Sick Children,
  Great Ormond Street, London

The Institute of Child Health
The Middlesex Hospital Medical
  School
The Royal Society of Medicine
St Mary's Hospital, Paddington,
  London
The Wellcome Institute of the
  History of Medicine
The World Health Organisation

Index